Beat Your Menopause Weight Gain

Balance Hormones, Stop Middle-Age Spread, Boost Your Health and Vitality

Silvana Siskov

Thank you for purchasing

Beat Your Menopause Weight Gain:
Balance Hormones,
Stop Middle-Age Spread,
Boost Your Health and Vitality

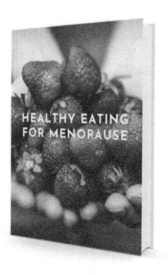

Please visit bit.ly/menopause-healthy-recipes
and download
Healthy Eating for Menopause – Recipe Book.

You will find plenty of delicious recipes there to
help you achieve a confident body.

BEAT YOUR MENOPAUSE WEIGHT GAIN:
BALANCE HORMONES, STOP MIDDLE-AGE SPREAD, BOOST YOUR HEALTH AND
VITALITY

www.silvanasiskov.com

Table of Contents

Introduction

Let's be honest; it is fabulous to be a woman, but it is not easy.

You are busy having fun when you are young and then suddenly your period comes along, shocking you to the core. Then, you just about get the hang of periods when they suddenly stop, signalling that there is a new life growing inside of you. Perhaps you are pregnant once, twice or maybe not at all, but then as you start to settle down, everything changes again and you begin to notice hot flushes, night sweats, weight gain, mood swings. Then, your period stops abruptly.

Yes, life as a woman is full of ups and downs and we have those pesky hormones to thank for it.

The fact you have picked up this book tells me that you are somewhere over the age of 40 and you are possibly wondering what is happening to your body. Do not worry, this happens to all of us and while reaching the age of menopause is not exactly a barrel of laughs, it is a natural part of every woman's life cycle.

The aim of this book is to help you through one of the most troublesome symptoms related to the menopause — weight gain. I know first-hand how difficult this phase of life can be. Not only are you experiencing changes within your body, but you are coming to terms with the fact that you are getting older and are no longer able to become pregnant. Though this is a natural part of the ageing process, it is a lot to take in and can be extremely traumatic for some women to handle.

The changes that the menopause can bring can easily affect the way you see yourself, the way you feel and your self-confidence, but it does not have to be such a negative experience. There are plenty of hints and tricks you can use to overcome some of the symptoms and effects this natural phase of life can bring.

Weight gain can be one of the most common and distressing parts of the menopause. By learning how to approach it positively, you can overcome the possible weight increase and successfully manage the other effects brought on by the menopause.

During this phase of your life, visceral fat is most common, leading to fat accumulations around the abdomen and collections around the internal organs. This increases your risk of developing serious health issues, such as type 2 diabetes, if left unchecked. Therefore, taking action is crucial. Apart from causing problems with your health, this also damages your confidence, because any type of weight gain can cause you to feel less than your best, sluggish and down.

Most women notice that as they enter the menopause, they start to gain weight more easily than before, and when they try to lose it, the entire process is much harder than it was in their earlier years. Not knowing the right ways to shift this fat can lead you to feel worse about yourself, which is not an enjoyable experience when combined with the other effects of the menopause.

Life is too short to spend time worrying and being upset about the menopause; you simply need to take advice and find ways to avoid or overcome the worst effects. That is where I can help.

I want to show you that while the menopause is inevitable, it does not need to be an end to your years of feeling beautiful, attractive and full of life. Those years can continue and become even better — once everything settles down. Remember, you are still the same strong and independent woman you were before the menopause arrived; it is just that a few bodily changes are happening that are causing you to feel a little less like yourself at present. However, this feeling will begin to change, and you will start to feel like yourself again.

The menopause can be a time for you to realise your power and use it as a springboard towards getting what you really want out of life. By focusing on health and well-being, you can feel better in yourself and open new doors of opportunity. Who knows what changes will come your way as a result of all this brimming confidence? You are giving yourself a chance to start over and do the things you never did before; it is a second chance to live your life to the full.

You do not have to deny yourself the things you enjoy to lose the menopause-related weight. You do not have to avoid looking in the mirror, and you do not have to think about your age and allow it to turn your mindset towards the negative end of the scale. Instead, why not let me show you the way forward? It is a decision you will not regret.

You will learn not only how to avoid menopausal weight gain and lose any weight you might have noticed creeping on, but also how to view the menopause as something that is just happening *to you*, not as something which is there to define you as a woman.

I know how you feel. I have been there myself and have helped countless women just like you to cope with this challenging yet surmountable time of life. All you need to do is keep an open mind, focus on the positive aspects of the menopause experience and read on.

Chapter 1

Perimenopause, Menopause, and Postmenopause — What Is It All About?

By reading and following the advice I give you in this book, not only will you learn to view the menopause through positive eyes, but you will also learn what you need to do to avoid the weight gain that so many women face around this period of life.

I will not lie and tell you that the menopause will be a breeze for all women. We are all unique in our own and extraordinary ways and that means there is never going to be a one size fits all answer to any health approach. Women have been going through what we affectionately call "the change" for centuries, so we are well placed to understand what is going on and learn from their experience and successfully overcome some of the challenging effects.

Perimenopause, Menopause, Postmenopause — What do These Terms Mean?

Before we delve into the finer details of the menopause, I must first arm you with the knowledge and understanding required. You need to understand what the terms I am going to use mean, i.e. perimenopause, menopause and postmenopause. Only then can you properly understand not only what I am talking about, but what it means for you.

This chapter is focusing on giving you basic but very important information about the three menopausal phases.

Before we delve into the main issue here, i.e. how to avoid menopausal weight gain, you need to have some background knowledge. You might already know something about the menopause through talking to other women or doing your own research, but for the sake of clarity, let's go through some of the basics.

Remember that information on the internet about anything health-related can be unreliable; anyone can publish information online, and it does not have to be fact-checked. However, you know that you can trust the information in this book and will not need to carry out any Google searches for clarification.

What Is the Difference Between the Perimenopause and the Menopause?

The perimenopause is the time before the actual menopause is established. During this time, you may experience a range of different symptoms. It is not unusual for periods to stop and start, or feel perfectly "normal" one day and be overwhelmed with the menopausal symptoms that can make you feel miserable or anxious the following day. Many women have mistakenly thought they were pregnant, only to find out later that they were perimenopausal, and vice versa.

In the following chapter, I am going to talk in more detail about the symptoms of the perimenopause and the menopause, as it is crucial to understand that during this period of a woman's life, hormonal imbalance can cause so many issues and can turn your life upside down. You will learn more about this as you read through this book.

The perimenopausal period, loosely translated as "around the menopause" can last for a few years. In some cases, it may last anything up to 10 years. This stage runs into the actual menopause itself when your periods stop entirely.

The first sign that you are perimenopausal and therefore heading towards the menopause comes in the shape of irregular periods. Your regular pattern may show changes, e.g. your periods might be lighter or heavier than before. You might start to have them more frequently or they can become less frequent and have no actual pattern. This can be extremely bothersome, as you have no way to predict when your period is due. Going away on holiday can be troublesome because you cannot plan when Mother Nature is going to come calling.

The perimenopause usually starts in a woman's forties, but in some cases it can begin earlier, in the late thirties. It is possible, though unusual, for some women to start in their twenties. There is no way of knowing when your particular menopausal period will start. There is some suggestion that you should look to your mother and when she began to go through her "change", but again, we are all unique, and that means there is no menopausal crystal ball for us to predict the start of the menopause. In my family, my mother had her last period around her 55th birthday. My sister is 55 now, and she is following in my mother's steps.

But my situation is very different — I had my last period at the age of 49. So, do we all need to look at our mothers to know when we will begin with the "change"? No. We can never know exactly when it will happen.

So, if the perimenopause is the time before the menopause, what is the actual menopause?

Menopause is easy to define — this is the point when your ovaries stop releasing eggs. At this stage, your periods will stop completely. You will no longer be able to get pregnant naturally, and your reproductive years are now behind you.

A Word about Postmenopause

Once the menopause is over, i.e. once you have not had a period for one full year (assuming you are 50 or over, and two full years if you are under 50), you enter the postmenopausal phase. As the name suggests, this is the time after you experienced the menopause, but that does not necessarily mean that all your symptoms will magically disappear.

It is not unusual for some women to continue to experience symptoms for up to 10 years afterwards. However, during this time the symptoms are usually a little less severe. They will begin to diminish gradually as time goes on, leaving you free to enjoy life without hot flushes and other annoying issues that the menopause can bring your way.

These uncomfortable symptoms occur because the former levels of oestrogen and progesterone have dropped, which is what caused the menopause in the first place.

The good news is that you will not have menstruation anymore, and the presence of periods in your life is now completely behind you. You will be able to enjoy greater freedom in all your activities such as going swimming at any time of the month. If you do notice any bleeding and you are definitely in the postmenopausal phase, you should see your doctor for a checkup.

You are Currently Being Controlled by Your Hormones

Hormones are extremely powerful, but we tend to underrate their influence on our body's functions. They help to regulate our weight (more on that shortly), mood, sleep, growth and a broad range of other tasks that add to our overall health and well-being. We need to look in more detail at the two main hormones controlling menopause;

they are called oestrogen and progesterone. Decreased levels of these two hormones during the menopause can cause many unpleasant symptoms.

These hormones are also connected to your menstrual cycle. However, as we become a little older, our levels of these hormones begin to drop. When this happens, our hormonal balance is totally out of sync, which is why you may experience a variety of symptoms during this time, such as mood swings or agitation.

Depending upon the severity of your symptoms, your doctor may suggest that you start Hormone Replacement Therapy (HRT) to help you balance your hormones. HRT effectively replaces the hormones that are low due to the approaching menopause. However, that is a choice that every woman must decide for herself and you should read about the pros and cons of this treatment before you make a final decision.

This book is not about treatment for the menopause. Therefore, I am not going to dwell on HRT. However, for the sake of clarity it has to be mentioned.

If you want to learn more about different menopausal symptoms and how to handle them, my book, *Free Yourself From Hot Flushes and Night Sweats: The Essential*

Guide to a Happy And Healthy Menopause might be an interesting read for you. In this book you will discover how to reduce your hot flushes and night sweats and find out about the effects of the menopause on your libido. You will learn many ways to deal with the menopause and its associated symptoms by making smart lifestyle changes, so you can approach the menopause with the right mindset.

If you are managing the effects of the menopause well and simply want to avoid weight gain, which is often one of the main factors affecting a woman's confidence and causing damage to her health, then the rest of this book will undoubtedly be of interest to you.

What you need to understand at this point is that hormones, or a lack thereof, control every aspect of your menopausal experience. This is a natural part of the ageing process for a woman and while it can be difficult to understand or deal with, take heart in the fact that it is normal.

It is easy to become scared or worried about what is happening to your body when you are starting to notice changes, but remember that you are simply going through a natural process. Recognising this should help you deal with any anxiety you experience and leave you free to focus on one burning topic….

Why Does All of This Lead to Weight Gain?

Ah, the very crux of this book!

Unfortunately, the hormonal ups and downs happening during the perimenopausal and menopausal stages mean that you will probably notice a little weight gain. During this time, most women see that they are putting weight on without even trying.

You are probably not eating anything different and you feel that you are not moving any less, but the scales begin to creep up a little. You will probably notice this particularly around your midriff; this is the visceral fat that I talked about in the introductory section.

There are two things to pay attention to here — firstly, the confidence issue. There are not many women who are happy to put on weight and simply live with it. It is bound to dent your confidence a little, especially if you are noticing extra pounds without having done anything to deserve it! Let's be honest, if you have been away on holiday and enjoyed the cakes and wine a little too much, you know that you are going to have to cut back when you get home, but if you have done nothing, to cause this change; it is quite a shock!

Weight gain can have an extremely damaging effect on the way you feel about yourself in general. Some women may have had a weight problem in the past, battled to lose it and felt proud of their efforts (rightly so), only to find that their hormones want to undo their hard work when the menopausal period begins. Quite understandably, this can be upsetting and extremely discouraging, affecting not only your confidence but also harming your self-worth.

The second important aspect is that visceral fat can be injurious to your health because it accumulates around the internal organs. This may increase the possibility of you developing chronic diseases and severe health conditions such as heart disease, diabetes, stroke, high blood pressure, high cholesterol levels and liver problems. These are just a few examples of serious health issues, which can damage your quality of life and may even prove to be fatal. We need to do everything we can to reduce these risk factors, to ensure that we all live long and healthy lives.

The problem is that this menopausal weight gain can be harder to shift than the weight gain from your younger age. For some reason, you put weight on more easily, yet it will not go away without a fight! It is surely one of life's rather unpleasant ironies.

By understanding why this is happening you can work out ways to overcome this problem, and I promise you, it can be beaten!

To understand it, let's delve a little deeper.

Many studies show that during the menopause the two main female sex hormones — oestrogen and progesterone, start fluctuating. Changes in these hormones can lead to developing excess weight around the middle.

During this time of your life, your testosterone levels will also decrease, leading to muscle mass loss. Testosterone is the male sex hormone but women have it too. When you lose muscle, your body will no longer be able to burn fat fast and you will gain weight easily. This happens naturally as you grow older and unless you are in the gym every day pumping iron (nobody has time for that), it is something you are certainly going to notice.

Hormonal imbalance during the menopause is known to cause increased appetite and higher calorie intake. Many women have higher fasting insulin levels and insulin resistance during this period of their lives. This can significantly affect the rate of their metabolism. It causes their metabolism to slow down, and this affects how fast they burn fat. The fact is, the slower you burn fat, the more fat you have; the quicker you burn fat, the less fat you have. A slower metabolism has an adverse effect on the function of the postmenopausal body.

In addition to regulating the menstrual cycle, oestrogen is a hormone which is also responsible for managing your weight and ensuring that your metabolism is functioning correctly. It impacts the amount of fat in the body.

As you move through the perimenopause and into the menopause, the slow decline of oestrogen (a type called estradiol in particular) can cause your body to store more fat. This results in weight gain and has a potentially harmful effect on bone density, leading to osteoporosis and poor heart health.

Hormonal imbalances caused by the menopause can affect your sleep quality, and if you are sleep deprived, you are more likely to make poor food choices and reduce the amount of exercise you are doing, simply because you are so tired. Lack of sleep will also affect your "hunger" hormones known as leptin and ghrelin. These two hormones are known to influence your hunger level and increase your appetite.

As you will learn later on in this book, sleep disruption is one of the menopause symptoms, so, yet again we have another trigger for the weight-increase to deal with.

However, do not despair, because I have plenty of advice on handling this problem and keeping your weight in check. What you need to do is to focus your time and attention on becoming healthier, eliminating unhealthy habits, and making good, firm, and positive choices instead.

Eating healthy and moving your body more are the two main good habits that can help control your menopausal weight gain, in addition to several other factors. In this book, we will explore some of those factors and look at what you need to do to achieve your weight loss goal.

Learning to See the Menopause From a Positive Perspective

If there is one thing I understand more than anything else on this subject, it is just how detrimental the menopause can be to some women's emotional health. It is a rollercoaster that you think will never end and while at the back of your mind you know that it will, in reality, it seems as though it will always be in your life, controlling your every move and every thought.

It has been quite a few years since I went through the "change", when I felt totally drained and overwhelmed by my menopausal symptoms, but I still remember thinking "I can't go through life feeling like this anymore". Since then, I have learnt a lot about the menopause and how to handle its symptoms. I wish I had known then what I know now. At the time I felt like it was never going to end, but remember this — you have control, you just need to take it back!

Putting on weight and noticing changes in your body, as well as the realisation that your reproductive years are coming to an end, can impact a woman's confidence levels. Lack of confidence can easily lead you down negative roads, such as turning to food or drinking too much to deal with the way this deficit makes you feel.

Emotional eating is often a choice that many women make to help them cope with their problems. The difficulty with seeking comfort in overeating is that it does not solve any problems. This impulsive behaviour usually makes the situation much worse than before.

Self-care is crucial during this time of your life. There are many healthy outlets for your emotions. It is vital that you look towards these, rather than overeating, smoking, or drinking too much. These coping devices will simply cause your weight to increase even more, further compounding your lack of confidence and making the entire problem much worse. When you think negatively, you feel negative; when you think positively and make positive life choices, you feel more positive and therefore much happier. This has a knock-on effect on every aspect of your life, your health included.

I suggest you speak to a friend, look for support networks in your local community, take your mind off what is going on within your body and instead look towards positivity. Yes, your body is changing, and yes, this does mean that you are no longer fertile, but hopefully, by this age, you were not thinking about having more children anyway. The thought of this is likely to make you shudder, but even if it does not, consider this your freedom card.

No more periods, no more PMS, the freedom to go swimming and stay in the water as long as you like and wear white as much as you like. These might seem like small things, but when you have spent a lifetime so far dealing with them, the freedom might be quite refreshing!

The menopause does not have to define you and it does not have to be a full stop to anything. It is merely something that is happening within your body, and with time you will simply go about your life as before, or perhaps with even more confidence as you realise your true capabilities.

Key Points

This has been an informational chapter to help you understand more about the perimenopausal phase and why it is different from the actual menopause. You were also introduced to the term "postmenopause".

You cannot learn how to handle and deal with something unless you realise what is going on and why. Hopefully, by this point, you have gained a clearer picture of what this time in your life is about, and you have realised that this is a normal process in every woman's life.

The aim of this book is to teach you how to avoid and reduce weight gain during the menopause and to educate you about the role of hormones and their influence on your weight.

The main points to remember from this chapter are:

- The perimenopause is the period before the actual menopause.

- Most women enter the perimenopause in their forties. However, this can be as early as their late thirties or even sooner in some cases.

- Every woman is unique.

- The menopause occurs when your ovaries no longer release eggs and you are therefore no longer fertile.

- The two critical female hormones are oestrogen and progesterone, and during this time, they begin to fall gradually.

- Hormones have a crucial role in regulating many different bodily functions, including sleep and metabolism.

- As oestrogen levels fall, your metabolism slows down. This can lead to weight gain as well as potentially affecting your sleep levels. Sleep deprivation can affect your "hunger" hormones and cause you to gain weight due to poor food choices.

- Weight gain during the menopause can be managed and overcome provided you make changes to your diet and lifestyle.

Chapter 2

Signs the Menopause is Around the Corner

Now that you know what the perimenopause and menopause are, we need to talk about the symptoms. This will help you to identify when this time of life is coming your way, or whether you might already be there.

Remember, every woman is different, which means you may experience all of the symptoms I am going to talk about, or you may only experience a few. You might be fortunate and barely experience any at all. The average woman could experience several common symptoms for up to a decade before the ovaries stop releasing eggs and the whole process is complete.

You might be slightly perturbed by the list of symptoms I am about to talk about, but remember that these can be mild, moderate, and rarely severe. If you are experiencing severe symptoms that affect your quality of life, consult your doctor and find out if any treatment options might help you cope a little better.

The other piece of good news is that this list of symptoms is unlikely to be constant. You might experience them on some days, most days for a month, and then none for a while. There is no way to predict how the menopause is going to impact you in terms of symptoms and severity, but it is vital to know what is normal and what is not.

Signs of the Perimenopausal Period

The most common signs that you are heading towards menopause, i.e. you are in the perimenopausal stage are the following:

- **Experiencing hot flushes** – Hot flushes are sudden and very short sensations of heat, which creep up your chest, into your neck and up to your face. You might also look flushed, i.e. a little red in the face, and you might even sweat. However, you might simply feel like you are red and sweaty but show no external signs at all. Some women suffer severely with hot flushes. They might get soaking wet within 10 seconds, but then they could spend the next 60 seconds freezing due to the changes in their body temperature.

- **Night sweats** – Alongside the hot flushes that usually occur while awake, you may also experience night sweats. These tend to wake you up unexpectedly and mimic the sensation of a hot flush. They disappear as quickly as they come, but by that point you are already awake, boiling hot, soaking wet and your night's sleep is disturbed. As soon as the night sweat disappears, you are freezing cold and searching for the extra blanket.

- **Sleep problems** – Aside from the night sweats, you may notice that you have difficulty nodding off to sleep at night, or you wake up frequently. This is due to the falling hormone levels, especially oestrogen, which affect your relaxation and sleep routine. As a result, you are likely to be irritable the next day and lack energy because you have missed out on a good night's sleep. You will most probably turn to sugary foods in order to regain your strength. The longer this cycle continues, the worse the next day symptoms become.

- **Vaginal dryness and discomfort** – This is caused by the falling hormone levels, which can cause vaginal dryness and discomfort during sex. This may sometimes lead to itching and soreness in the vaginal area, and some women notice that they also experience more yeast infections during this time. If you notice these symptoms, try using a lubricant during sex to make the experience more comfortable and to avoid soreness.

- *More urinary tract infections (UTIs)* – Some women are more prone to UTIs than others. If you notice you are experiencing more of these rather irritating occurrences during the perimenopausal period than before, a consultation with your doctor is necessary.

- *Issues with concentration and forgetfulness* – Many women notice that they suddenly develop a case of "baby brain" – without the baby – during this time. We can blame hormones once more here, but it could also be due to the lack of sleep.

- *Experiencing palpitations* – Falling oestrogen levels or fluctuations during the perimenopause can often lead to palpitations. During palpitations your heart will be pounding and beating fast for a few seconds. You must remain calm if you experience these. Practising yoga and meditation are known to be great for making you feel more relaxed which can help with palpitations. I advise you to visit your doctor if you experience this problem regularly. Keep in mind that changes in hormone levels are typically connected to increased palpitations.

- *Headaches* – Headaches are another side effect of your hormones being totally out of sync at this time. However, if you have severe headaches or migraines, do consult your doctor; it might have nothing to do with the menopause!

- *Weight gain* – The very subject of this book. Reduced muscle mass resulting in weight gain is one of the most common complaints from menopausal women, and we already know that visceral fat can be dangerous. Many women also notice a change in their general body shape at this time. By focusing on lifestyle changes, which I will discuss as we move through the coming chapters, you will be more in control of managing your weight during the menopause.

Remember, just because you are not experiencing *all* of the symptoms above, it does not mean there is anything wrong; every woman is different.

When Is the Menopause Over?

How will you know when you finished with the menopause and the postmenopause started?

Good question!

It is easy to say you have completed the menopause once you feel yourself again and are no longer experiencing symptoms, but those pesky hormones might not have got the memo. There may be fluctuations in your hormone levels after the menopause is over. If that does happen, the symptoms are likely to be mild and possibly unnoticeable.

I have already mentioned and it is worth mentioning again — you are considered postmenopausal after your periods have stopped entirely for two years if you are under the age of 50 and for one year if you are over the age of 50. That means no periods for one or two years straight, depending upon your age. By that time, you will also notice that most of the symptoms have reduced or disappeared. A few women experience severe symptoms for some years, but this is unusual, and most return to their normal self shortly after entering the postmenopause.

The postmenopause may bring its own challenges; there is no phase in a woman's life free of challenges, but the perimenopausal stage seems to affect women's well-being the most. A variety of unpleasant symptoms that we face during this period is something that many women struggle with. Some women argue that the menopause is the most difficult time of their lives due to experiencing physical symptoms and going through psychological and emotional changes, which affect their health, confidence and general well-being.

Let's explore this further in the next section.

How the Menopause May Affect Your Confidence?

The menopause is not just about the physical symptoms you are experiencing; it is also about how it makes you feel about yourself. Never underestimate just how important your confidence is in life — it affects a whole range of areas: your motivation to make changes to your relationships, self-worth and a host of other unexpected things. Self-confidence in life is key, and it can be affected by the smallest thing.

Whenever we go through significant life changes, it is easy to be knocked off-kilter and experience a minor confidence crisis. Some women sail through the menopause, but more tend to struggle a little with confidence at some stage. You are not alone if you are struggling with the menopause. Never feel that you simply have to woman up and deal with it; this is a big issue in your life and you need to progress through it in a way that feels right to you and to find support from those around you.

It is normal to be affected by this massive change in life, but that does not mean that you should dwell on the negatives. Every woman has a different symptom that causes them the most trouble. For some, it could be the lack of energy and tiredness, due to those fluctuating hormones. For others, it could be weight gain, or it could be feeling agitated. The entire cocktail of hormonal effects leaves you open to potential mood changes, and it can also drastically affect the way you think of yourself inside. This is likely to cause you to feel a different sense of self. Your confidence will take a hit as a result, because you may have developed a different perspective.

Many women start to worry that they are no longer attractive, but the truth is that a menopausal woman is no less and no more beautiful than a woman who is yet to go through the menopause. Whether or not you are able to menstruate has no bearing on your beauty both inside or out! Look at some of the sexiest stars in the celebrity world, perhaps Jennifer Lopez, as one example — she is over 50, and she is undoubtedly still attractive and sexy! Attractiveness and sexiness have nothing to do with your ability to carry a child, your ability to menstruate and certainly nothing to with your ability to release an egg from your ovaries every month!

You are just as beautiful as you were before you started the menopause, and that is not going to change because of your hormones. Once the menopause is over, many women reclaim their confidence to the point where they never look back. There is nothing sexier or more attractive than a woman who is comfortable in her body, owning her sexuality and someone who exudes confidence in who she is. That is a cocktail for real confidence and happiness right there! It does not matter how old or young she is, or whether she is menopausal or not. What matters is the way she feels about herself.

However, I want you to know that if you do feel a little lacking in confidence at this stage of your life, it is entirely normal. Many women feel this way, and there is nothing wrong with you if you are not feeling your very best. Life changes can knock us sideways sometimes, and hormones are powerful things. It is not easy to battle hormones every single day and get up and go about your business at the same time. You should pat yourself on the back for having the power to do just that. All you need to do is carry on doing what you are doing for a little longer, with perhaps a few changes to your outlook and lifestyle to battle any weight gain issues.

Of course, emotions are just as powerful as hormones. If you are genuinely struggling, seek help from your loved ones, look for support networks of women who are also going through the same time in life as you, or have a chat with your doctor if you are feeling low. There is help out there, and even though feeling down and lacking in confidence at this stage of life is quite common, you do not have to live with it.

Before I end this chapter, it is important to mention that the lifestyle changes I will discuss throughout the rest of the book will go a long way to giving you back your power and, therefore, your confidence. When you take ownership of your health and your body, you step into your power. This fuels your confidence and helps you to understand just how strong you really are.

Key Points

There is a range of symptoms that signal you are in the menopausal period of your life, but it is vital to remember that every woman is different, so you might not experience all of them or even many of them. Symptoms can vary in severity too, so if you are particularly struggling with one symptom, seek help from your doctor to find ways to reduce its effect on your life.

Women find the main issue with the menopause is often not the symptoms, but the effects that it can have on their confidence. The idea of going through the menopause can easily cause a woman to feel bad about herself, and when you add to the mix weight gain and sleep deprivation, the whole thing can become a rather unpleasant experience. The good news is that throughout this book, I am going to give you actionable, easy to follow advice on how to reduce the effects, thereby helping you to look and feel your best throughout the menopause and beyond.

The main points to remember from this chapter are:

- You have completed the menopause when you have had no periods for two years straight if you are under the age of 50, or one year if you are over this age.

- Menopausal symptoms can range in severity, from mild to severe.

- Every woman will experience a different combination of symptoms.

- If you struggle with symptoms, it is important to seek help to reduce their effects.

- The menopause itself can easily affect a woman's confidence, especially if she gains weight.
- Fluctuations in hormones can cause havoc with how you feel, so it is vital to take it easy on yourself.

- You are just as beautiful *now* as you were *before* the menopause — the menopause does not dictate your beauty or your worth.

Chapter 3

Stress, Weight Gain and the Menopause

How many times per day do you utter the words "I am so stressed?" and how many times do you hear other people around you saying it?

Probably a lot.

We tend to say we are stressed most of the time when the reality is that we are not. We do not take stress as seriously as we should. Did you know that stress can be life-threatening when left to grow over the long term? It sounds dramatic, but it is true. You will come to realise how, as I talk more about why it is dangerous and what detrimental impact stress can have. However, a little pressure can be useful because it serves as a motivator.

Confused?

Do not be.

A little stress is useful in some cases, but when stress is allowed to build up and last over a long period, it can be extremely damaging. It can damage your mental and physical state.

How does this link to the menopause?

Menopause can be a stressful time for a woman. If you are struggling with menopausal symptoms, unhappy with weight gain, and generally feeling low in confidence and mood, the stress will easily creep into your life and cause everything to seem so much more strenuous and hard to cope with.

Everyone has been through a period of real stress at some point in their lives. Can you remember how it felt for you? You probably could not concentrate for very long and you might have had trouble sleeping. Maybe you even turned to overeating or adopted another damaging way to handle the emotions you were experiencing? You probably snapped at everyone in your close vicinity and might have ended up having arguments for no reason whatsoever.

It is common to feel more stress at this time of your life, simply because you might be lacking in sleep, you feel confused or worried about what is going on inside your body (or in your life in general), your hormones are all over the place, and everything seems a little out of control. You may be experiencing brain fog too, and your memory does not seem to be as sharp as it used to be. While going through the menopause can itself cause weight gain, surprisingly so can stress. That means that managing a healthy weight could be even more difficult than when you are younger.

It is common for menopausal women to face many stressful events in addition to the changes they experience inside their bodies. Stressful events that are most prevalent for women in their forties and fifties are associated with children leaving home, going through a divorce, or taking care of elderly parents. Any of these events can bring a tremendous amount of stress.

In this chapter, I am going to talk to you about what stress is and the stress hormone that might join the mix and cause even more difficulties during the menopause. I will finish off by discussing how you can do your best to reduce the amount of stress you have in your life.

You must learn to handle stress healthily. Enough is going on in your life as things stand; you do not need extra worry and problems.

So, first things first, let's talk about what stress is.

Fight or Flight? The Dangers of Stress and the Role of Cortisol

Before I can explain why stress causes weight gain, I need to explain the stress process.

Stress is an emotion, but it is also a process and a reaction. To understand it, we need to go back to the days of cavemen and cavewomen. In that era, there were a million and one things to run away from. These included terrifying beasts who were trying to eat them. Of course, we do not have these problems to worry about nowadays, thankfully, but the human brain has not evolved since then on the stress front. I am talking about the "fight or flight" response here.

In those days, our ancestors would experience a fight or flight reaction to either turn towards the threat and fight it or run away from it. Those were the only two options.

The human brain is always on the lookout for a threat; something that is going to threaten our safety and well-being. That is why humans are hard-wired to be negative before they are positive; the brain is on safety mode most of the time.

So, while your brain is trying to keep you safe, it also perceives situations to be threatening when, in reality, they are not. When the brain decides that something is a threat, it kickstarts the stress process and gets the body ready to either fight it or run away from it. Extra endorphins are released to help you out in this situation, additional oxygen is available and a stress hormone cortisol is released.

Let's look at two examples now. In case number one, you face a real threatening situation. For example, a dangerous animal is about to attack you. What will you do? There are two options — you will run away from the threat or fight it and win, and the whole thing will be over. You will be affected by this and feel tired for a short while, but then you will be fine. Your hormonal levels will return to normal and your body will stop pumping out cortisol until the next time the brain recognises a threat.

In the second example, there is no real threat, and the brain has got it wrong. You have not fought something or run away from anything, but the brain is scanning the environment —worrying — and remains stuck in the stress zone. What does this mean? It means your body is on high alert and the cortisol is running loose around your body. You see, this is the situation we find ourselves in most of the time. We are sometimes late for an important meeting, worried about paying bills, going through a divorce, etc. These situations can cause stress, and our body will react to each of them as if we are facing a real danger.

When left to run wild in this situation, stress is damaging. In the first example, we face a real dangerous situation, and our body reacts to it accordingly. That is perfectly fine. It is what the body is supposed to do. However, the second example is not healthy. Unfortunately, it is a situation that is all too common in the fast-paced and demanding world we live in today.

So, what do high levels of cortisol do that is so damaging? The answer is — many things, but in the context of this book, it makes you put on weight. Several studies suggest that chronically raised cortisol levels contribute to increased insulin in the blood. This is one of the main contributors to weight gain as insulin controls the blood glucose level, which converts food energy into fat. We must not ignore the fact that raised cortisol level often causes cravings for sweets, high-fat and salty foods. Apart from contributing to the elevated insulin levels, these foods are also known to lead to poor health, low energy levels, and weight gain.

It is important to mention that when entering the perimenopausal stage, the decreased level of oestrogen tends to increase the cortisol level. Therefore, it is even more important to follow some basic self-care principles which include a plant-based diet and a healthy lifestyle. Your health and well-being depend on how much effort you put into taking proper care of your body.

As I have already mentioned, the menopause is a stressful time for many women and because you might experience its symptoms for anything up to 10 years, that is a long time for stress to be present in someone's body. While the lack of muscle mass can cause weight gain during this time, stress also adds to the situation and compounds it further.

As well as raising insulin, another reason for cortisol causing weight gain is that it stimulates the metabolism and demands from energy to come thick and fast. It is doing this because it is part of the stress reaction, i.e. the fight or flight response. It needs the energy to run or fight, even when there is nothing to fight with or run away from. In this situation, the body wants the energy quickly and tends to search for it from high-fat foods and carbs. A red light should be flashing straight away because those are two food groups that can certainly cause weight gain when used in the wrong way. And not only that but these foods are also damaging to your health. They cause inflammation in the body and can lead to serious diseases.

All of this stimulates the release of insulin, which then affects your overall blood sugar levels. Therefore, it is no surprise that a long period of stress can be a contributing risk factor for the development of diabetes over the long term. In effect, you will crave foods that are sweet, high in fat and therefore high in sugar and quite salty. These foods will cause you to pile on the pounds if you eat them too often, which you probably will if you are feeling too stressed over a more extended period.

So to conclude, cortisol is not your friend, and especially not during the menopause.

Why Is Stress so Common During the Menopause?

I have already mentioned this in passing, but let's discuss it further for clarity's sake.

I should point out that not every woman is going to feel stressed during the menopause. Some women do not feel stressed at all, others feel it occasionally and some women find their stress levels are continually high over this period. It is a personal experience that might differ from someone else's, but it is a time when you are more likely to notice issues and become more upset about them.

Many people struggle with changes in their lives, but it is hard to get away from it when the change is occurring within your body. This can cause anxiety. The more you sit and worry about it, the more stress is going to build up. If your menopausal symptoms are causing your lack of sleep, this is a significant precursor for stress once more.

You might also find that you are agitated and short tempered with your partner or the people around you. If this causes ructions within your relationships and friendships, you are again creating a stressful situation.

It is essential to mention that finding the right strategies to cope with stress in your life is as important as finding proper ways to manage stress inside your body. These two types of stress are closely connected and significantly affect one another. Their relationship impacts how you react to stressful situations you experience in life and any problem you face regularly.

There are countless reasons why the menopause might be a high-stress period for a woman, but the good news is that it is manageable when you educate yourself and learn how to change your mindset towards the positive. It is vital that you avoid unhealthy coping mechanisms, such as overeating, spending too much money on shopping treats, drinking too much alcohol, smoking, using drugs or spending countless hours watching Netflix. You need to focus your mind on healthy coping methods and as I will highlight in the next section, there are plenty of these that will help you deal with stress levels, but also aid your menopausal symptoms.

It is easy to say repeatedly that there is nothing to worry about concerning the menopause, that you are no less of a woman because of this process and that perhaps you are more of a woman because you have got your badge to prove it! However, if you are feeling confused, if you are struggling with specific symptoms, or you are just not having the best of times when it comes to the perimenopausal or menopausal period of your life, no amount of reassurances will make a difference. In this case, you need to get practical, and that is what I am going to talk about in this next section.

10 Stress Management Techniques to Try Today!

Finding ways to deal with stress will not magically make the menopause end, or get it over and done with, but will make the entire process easier and possibly make your life far more fulfilling and enjoyable to live as a result.

The good news is, stress management techniques are not too difficult, and anyone can do them. You simply need to choose the ones which work best for you. However, it is a good idea to give them all a try and figure it out from there — you never know what is going to work and what is not until you have tried it for yourself.

Let's check out the 10 stress management techniques that you can start today.

Talk About the Problem

You might not have a specific issue causing the stress, but you may generally be feeling stressed out. That is quite a common feeling for a woman going through the menopause because the whole situation feels out of control, or specific symptoms are too troublesome. In that case, find someone you trust, perhaps someone who is also going through the menopause or has already gone through it, and talk about it. Talking to a qualified counsellor is always a good option. A counsellor can help you find your unique way of expressing your feelings and managing your emotions about the situation you are currently facing.

It does not matter what you say to the person you chose to share your worries and concerns. Whether it is a trusted friend or a counsellor, tell them whatever comes into your mind. Just get it out there. Talk about how you feel, the things that worry you, and the nagging doubts in the back of your mind.

The more you empty your brain of things which are concerning you, the lighter you will feel. Most people find that when they talk about something, it helps put it into perspective. Offloading your thoughts and feelings can be incredibly cathartic. Seeing a counsellor and finding your voice can help you to see and feel about things differently. It can take the burden off your shoulders and bring positivity into your life.

If you are struggling with your weight loss or feeling upset about the weight gain, talk about it with someone you trust and perhaps put a weight loss plan together. Find a friend you can exercise with or join a class; this is motivating and will give your workout a social element.

Spend More Time Outdoors

Mother Nature perhaps is not treating you very well right now, but she also has lots of natural healing to send your way too — head outside!

Sunlight and fresh air can help to reduce stress, anxiety and depression, allowing you to feel more uplifted and lighter on your feet. When you are feeling low or worried about something, a short time breathing in the fresh air outside can help to distract you and take your worries away. You are also benefiting from the increased vitamin D from the sunlight which is linked to increased mood; a lack of vitamin D during the winter months is associated with low mood.

Serotonin is another naturally occurring hormone within the body. It has positive effects. It regulates your mood and helps with sleep, memory and feelings of happiness. Being outdoors and in the sunlight can boost your serotonin levels. This can help to achieve a more upbeat mood which, as a result, decreases your stress levels.

Get Plenty of Exercise

This particular stress management technique is ideal for menopausal weight gain problems because it helps to battle that specific issue, alongside a healthy diet.

Exercise has many benefits. It can support your weight loss as well as help you feel less stressed. Exercising is known for boosting the mood and distracting your mind. Working out is excellent stress relief. During exercise, the body produces endorphins in your brain. These chemicals act as natural painkillers and support your well-being. They can also help you to sleep.

You can choose any exercise you like, but some are incredibly helpful for protecting the body against potential bone density loss, which contributes to osteoporosis in women over the menopausal age.

Try activities such as swimming, yoga or Pilates, as these are strength-building exercises which are also very low impact and easy to do. They help with breathing and this can reduce stress levels and improve sleep. Pilates moves are excellent for stretching and this helps with flexibility and balance. Swimming is perfect because you are surrounded by water, which is naturally calming. Yoga is another excellent choice because it teaches you to focus on your breathing and that in itself can help you overcome stressful situations when they occur.

Meditate and Try Mindfulness

Many women find meditation very useful when they feel stressed out, so this is certainly something you could try. The downside is that many women also struggle with meditation and give up too soon — this is something that takes time and practice, but the benefits are far-reaching once it is mastered. Quietening the mind can be difficult when there is so much going on, but it is possible with practice.

Try this:

- Choose a time when you will not be disturbed; turn your phone off and close the curtains.

- Sit or lay down somewhere comfortable.

- Close your eyes and turn your attention to your breathing.

- Breathe in slowly and steadily through your nose for the count of five.

- Hold the breath for a count of three.

- Slowly exhale through your mouth for a count of five.

- Repeat until you feel calm.

- If any thoughts try to enter your mind, simply acknowledge them and push them away.

- Keep focusing on your breathing until you have successfully managed to quieten the noise in your mind.

- Try and build up the amount of time you stay in the meditation exercise as you go along, but do not rush it.

- When you are ready, tell yourself that you are going to open your eyes and slowly do so, staying seated or laid down for a few minutes until you are feeling more alert.

You can try countless meditation types, but many women find guided group meditations to be very useful. You could seek out groups of women who are also going through this time in their lives and join in. This will allow you to meet new friends in the same situation as you and help banish your stress at the same time.

Something else you can try is mindfulness. This can be particularly useful when dealing with life changes that are the very crux of your stress. Mindfulness teaches you to live in the present moment and not to worry about the past or think too far into the future. That is something all of us could do with trying more!

Many women tend to think back over the past and their fertile years, perhaps comparing how they looked and felt back then to how they look and feel after menopausal weight gain. Being overweight can cause some women to feel unattractive. Also, excess weight can negatively impact our health and energy levels. It can be very easy to look back and make yourself feel bad about these changes. Similarly, you might be thinking too far into the future, worrying about what comes next and how you are going to deal with becoming a little older.

Using mindfulness can help push all of this to one side and help you to focus on you in the here and now. Also, meditation, reading inspiring books, and having regular contact with people who lift your spirit can significantly increase your confidence and improve the way you feel about yourself.

Again, it can be hard to do but you need to stick with it and practice, without trying to rush things. An excellent way to start is to head outside for a walk. Leave your phone at home or keep it on silent in your bag, and make sure that your attention is firmly on the place you are in right now, e.g. the road, the field, the park, the beach, or wherever else you are. Be in the here and now. Enjoy the moment!

Walk along at a slow pace if you can, and try the breathing exercise I mentioned a few paragraphs ago. Of course, keep your eyes open! Once you are calm enough, turn your attention to your surroundings. Notice the vibrant green of the leaves on the tree; really tune into them and notice how the sunlight glints off them, or how the wind gently blows them around.

Once you have taken in every element of that tree, slowly, turn your attention to something else, perhaps the clouds in the sky or the dog running around in the field next to you.

By being absorbed in the current moment, you keep your mind in the here and now, distracting yourself from unhelpful and stressful thoughts. Over time, you are going to notice a greater appreciation of what is around you and will not be bothered by petty worries half as much as you used to be. This is ideal for stress management, but it is also a great way to live.

Focus on Your Sleep

Focusing on your sleep is the key. It has such a powerful effect on your health and quality of life. Lack of sleep can be one of the menopausal symptoms and having problems with sleep can worsen stress. Therefore, focusing on improving the quality and duration of sleep is vital.

Easier said than done, yes, but totally possible.

If you are regularly struggling with sleep and feel you might have insomnia, it is a good idea to consult your doctor and see if anything can be done about this issue. However, most of the time, making some simple changes to your sleeping routine and implementing a few useful tips can help you to have a better quality sleep.

I will not go into too much detail here, as I am going to cover a whole chapter on the connection between sleep and weight loss a little later on. For now, however, simply know that you need to focus on getting the best night's sleep possible on a regular basis to avoid stress and keep your weight steady and consistent. Of course, you will also feel far better in yourself if you are rested and alert, compared to feeling tired and agitated. It is very easy to allow worries and stress to overwhelm you when you feel this way.

Remember, good quality sleep is a very powerful medicine. And it is one of the best habits to implement in your everyday life to achieve good health and successful weight loss, in addition to a healthy diet and regular exercise.

Focus on Your Enjoyment

What do you like to do in your spare time? Whatever it is, do more of it!

It is very easy to focus your time on everyone and everything else: work, family, children, friends — a long to-do list, and most women do not spend enough of their time on themselves. It is not selfish to focus on yourself occasionally. It is actually necessary for your overall health and well-being, and extremely useful for excluding stress from the equation.

If you love to lay in a bath and read a book, do it. If you like to go shopping with a friend, go for it, as long as you are not spending money to mask your emotional upset, of course. If you enjoy crafts, baking, cooking, playing sports, pampering yourself, or simply sitting and watching the world go by, you have permission to do it. It is necessary and it is advisable.

Be Sociable and Do not Hide Yourself Away

When you are not feeling your best self or perhaps feeling a little low about how you look (just because you have gained a few pounds) and stressed out about everything around you, menopause included, it is easy to hide away and avoid social situations. I advise you not to do this!

Get out there, live your life, focus on having fun and you will find that stress quickly leaves your life as a result. You will also find the confidence within yourself to handle whatever the menopause has thrown at you. If you are going out with friends in the same age group as you, it is likely they are going to be experiencing the same or similar issues as you. I remember having long conversations with female friends about how menopausal symptoms affected our lives. Oh, I so wish I knew back then what I know about coping mechanisms now.

Being involved in the conversation on the topic of menopause with other women can sometimes lead to plenty of laughter. Sharing the misery of the menopause usually creates a light-hearted atmosphere and can put women in a much better mood. *A problem shared is a problem halved*, they say. So, if you can find someone who can relate to your problem, it lightens the mood.

Try Visualisation

Many women find visualisation a useful tool for stress management, but it can be used for several other problems too, such as negative thinking or simply when you need the motivation to get something done. If you feel stressed out, worried, or just focused on the negative side of things, turn your attention to how you want something to work out. This is a time when you *are* allowed to think of the future because you are doing it through positive eyes and not worried ones.

Sit somewhere quiet and close your eyes. Focus on your breathing until you have calmed your mind. When you are ready, picture how you want things to look, for instance, how you want to feel and how you want your future life to be. The more you picture it and add in details, the more real and effective it will be when you call the picture to your mind during a period of stress.

Of course, make sure that the picture you are visualising is realistic. It will not help if you picture yourself as a size zero on a beach in two months; if you are overweight right now, this is simply not realistic and probably not something that will make you truly happy anyway. It is far better to focus yourself on being happy, healthy and body confident. Visualisation will help you take actionable steps and pull you towards transformation with a much more powerful force.

Try Reframing Your Thoughts to Become More Positive

Stress happens far more readily when your mindset is generally negative. You may be feeling low because you are not happy with your appearance or struggling with menopausal symptoms. In this case, you need to try and focus on becoming more positive overall. By doing that, you will notice that your stress reduces, you have a new-found strength to overcome difficult emotions and you are able to look at life with a glass-half-full mentality.

Of course, changing your mindset in this way is not easy and may take a while to complete the process. Despite this, it is a very worthwhile way to spend your time.

Reframing is a cognitive behaviour therapy treatment method that seeks to change a person's mindset from negative to positive and can help with a wide range of different problems.

There is no reason why you cannot use it in this situation.

The downside of reframing is that you need to be continually aware of your thoughts at the start, and that is pretty tiring and time-consuming. Again, it is worthwhile. Stress will find it harder to overtake your life if you think more positively.

Try this:

- The next time you recognise that you are thinking something negative, acknowledge it as being negative.

- Think of something positive to counteract that negative thought. For instance, if you are thinking "My body is changing and I do not like it", change it to "How my body changes make me understand its power". You can use any example you want; this is just one of them.

- Then, repeat the positive thought several times, and try your best to visualise it too. If you can, say it aloud, as this will be more powerful and more useful to you.

- Repeat this with every negative thought you recognise.

Focus on Your Diet

We will dedicate a whole chapter to diet in a short while, so I will not dwell on the finer details here. However, when you are eating healthily — feeding your body with the right amounts of carbs, protein and fat, and getting all the vitamins and minerals you need — you can manage your weight more effectively as a result. You are going to be more upbeat and confident in yourself. That is a picture which stress will find difficult to creep into. We can compare this to putting the correct type of fuel into your car. If you fill the tank with the wrong fuel, it might damage your engine, and your vehicle will not be going anywhere.

When you feel stressed, you are also more likely to reach for unhealthy food choices as a way of coping. You know how it goes: you say to yourself, "I deserve a slice of chocolate cake, I have been so stressed out lately", but one slice leads to two or three, and then you start beating yourself up internally for not being more careful with your food choices. Of course, those slices of chocolate cake usually go straight to your hips, and as I have mentioned already, menopausal weight gain is far harder to lose *now* than previously.

61

Of course, this does not mean you cannot have the odd treat, or that you have to deny yourself everything you enjoy. It is all about moderation. That is key to achieving success with your health and weight loss goals, and we are going to look at it in the following chapter.

Key Points

This chapter has talked about the dangers of stress and how the menopause can be an incredibly stressful time for women. When left unchecked and allowed to grow, stress can be fatal. However, stress is something we all deal with in small amounts. Learning to handle stress by using stress management techniques is a vital part of the whole menopausal process. By mastering these, you will find that your menopausal story is far more comfortable to manage as a result.

The main points to remember from this chapter are:

- Stress can be extremely damaging to health when allowed to build up and remain in place for an extended period.

- The menopause can cause stress to a woman simply because her hormones are running wild, or she might be struggling to deal with the symptoms in general.

- The stress process is often referred to as "fight or flight".

- Much of the time, the brain misjudges what a real threat is, and as a result, the stress process kickstarts for no reason.

- During the stress reaction, the body releases a cortisol hormone, which can lead to weight gain over time.

- Learning to handle stress will allow you to be healthier, happier, and help you control your weight more successfully.

Chapter 4

Healthy Diet 101

Handling stress and approaching the menopause with a positive mindset is only part of the deal. Hormones may stimulate weight gain, but the food you put into your body will most likely cause you to gain weight at the end of the day.

The hormones might cause you to feel hungrier and make you less firm to resist food cravings, but if you are putting healthy foods into your body and focus on quality, you are far less likely to put weight on even if you consume more food than you require.

But do you know what a healthy diet is?

Many people falsely believe that a healthy diet means restriction and not being able to eat what you want. In truth, that is a fad diet and those types of diets do not work! If you are always on a fad diet, you will probably end up eating more in the end because the foods you eat will not satisfy you, and you will be fed up with not enjoying your favourite foods now and again, so you will rebel against it.

In this chapter, I am going to talk about what a healthy diet is, and what it is not. Of course, even if you stick to healthy food options and avoid going towards the unhealthier ones, you will still have to occasionally battle with your hormones, but remember one word throughout it all — moderation.

Moderation is key!

That means you can enjoy the odd slice of pizza, the occasional bar of chocolate, or the occasional glass of wine and it is totally fine and even encouraged, as long as the rest of your diet is healthy. Besides a nutritious diet, you should also make sure that you exercise regularly, but we will go over that in more detail shortly. Focusing on what is right for your body 80% of the time is all you need to do.

Remember, a healthy diet needs to be part of your lifestyle and not something you only do for a short while. If you want to avoid and rectify menopausal weight gain, you need to dedicate time to making life changes. So, in this case, moderation is going to be the one thing that you must apply to your new lifestyle. This will prevent you from making it so difficult for yourself that it is impossible to stay on track.

What does moderation look like?

It means you have a slice of pizza when you fancy and not the whole pizza. You have a glass of wine instead of the entire bottle, and you only have it once or twice a week. Even if you want alcoholic drinks every night, choose which two days you want to have them, and you stick to your decision. You have a few squares of chocolate rather than devouring a family-sized bar, or you have a takeaway once a week and not every night.

Moderation means you have a little of what you want, but in ways which mean it does not ruin your entire healthy lifestyle outlook.

You Really are What You Eat

We have all heard the saying, *You are what you eat*. This is true in so many ways and I agree to it. If you regularly eat processed meals and sugary snacks, and load up on sugary drinks every day, you will notice that your health suffers. Your health and weight will be affected by unhealthy eating and poor drinking habits.

Your skin will break out, your hair will lack shine, perhaps you will feel tired and sluggish, your sleep might be affected at night due to indigestion or the blood sugar crash, and of course, you are going to notice your clothes becoming a little tighter.

On the other hand, if you eat a healthy diet, you are healthier on the inside, and it shows on the outside. Your skin will glow, your hair will shine, your nails will be stronger and you will have more energy. You will be positive as a result of how you feel, and you will notice that you not only lose weight, but you maintain your ideal weight once you hit it. Your clothes will fit better, you will feel lighter on your feet and overall, you will simply feel more confident as a result of the physical effects.

So, if you eat poorly, you are unhealthy. If you eat well, you are healthy.

The foods you eat determine how healthy your body is going to be.

The problem with menopausal weight gain is that it can happen quickly and without warning. If your diet is not healthy to begin with, you are going to find that shifting the excess weight is an uphill battle. If you are eating healthily to start with, you might have the cravings that your hormonal imbalances cause, but if you have the right mindset, you will not have a major problem to deal with because you will not be reaching for unhealthy food choices.

The bottom line is that menopausal weight gain comes down to the ability to handle temptation. Your hormones are going to make you want to eat and they are going to turn their attention towards the worst types of foods. The hunger hormone is on the rampage and the satiety hormone, which responsibility is to reduce your appetite, has somehow disappeared. Giving in makes you feel worse in yourself, so you just eat more to make yourself feel better. It is such a vicious circle that so many women fall foul of, and before they realise it, they are faced with weight gain which takes a tremendous amount of effort to lose.

Hormones are potent, and you should never underestimate their ability to make you want to eat everything in the fridge or kitchen cupboards. You should also never underestimate how overwhelming the cravings can be. However, if you are hooked on the right types of food, the damage will be minimal, if at all.

So, while you are what you eat, if what you are eating is healthy, you do not have so much of a problem to begin with.

The Key Nutrients You Need Daily

During the menopause, as we have already explored, oestrogen and progesterone levels begin to decline. This can detrimentally affect your metabolism. It is important to ensure that your diet is therefore focused on health and well-being rather than towards enjoyment of all the processed and sugary foods the world likes to throw at us.

A healthy diet consists of macronutrients and micronutrients.

Macronutrients include:

- Protein

- Carbohydrate

- Fat

Micronutrients include:

- Vitamins

- Minerals

Do not be afraid to eat fats; simply make sure that you opt for the healthier versions. You need to look towards monounsaturated and polyunsaturated fats as a rule of thumb. Avoid trans fat as much as possible. This type of fat damages your health and causes weight gain.

Apart from macronutrients, you also need a range of different micronutrients, such as magnesium, potassium, zinc, iron, calcium and vitamins (A, B, C, D, E, etc.). These are important for the optimal health of your body.

To keep your body healthy, stick to eating whole organic foods as often as possible. These foods store beneficial nutrients that give your body energy and help to support and ensure the functioning of your main organs. Weight gain is a complicated process and can be put down to a range of different causes. When you feed your body with healthy foods and focus on portion sizes — not too much and not too little — you have a chance of maintaining a healthy weight. Of course, it is also essential to pay attention to your lifestyle and make sure you focus on implementing healthy choices as much as you can.

To ensure that your body receives all the essential nutrients needed for its healthy functioning, you should get the majority of your calories from foods such as fresh fruits and fresh vegetables, legumes, protein (lean), nuts and whole grains. When you consume too many foods or beverages that are high in trans fat and calories, e.g. fizzy drinks, chocolate or ice cream, you are not doing your body any favours and it is a recipe for weight gain!

The problem is, when your hormones are playing havoc with your metabolism, your body is automatically going to start craving the foods and drinks which are high in fat and sugar. Those foods can be detrimental to your health.

There are different types of diets. Some of them are focused mainly on counting calories. Others involve fasting and focusing on restricting daily eating windows. The popular Keto diet tends to be more focused on cutting back on carbs and increasing fats' consumption. In this book, I am not promoting any particular diet; I just want to outline a healthy diet as simply as possible to help you understand what you should be aiming for, versus what you should not. Understanding what a healthy diet includes and what your body requires, will help you decide what type of diet is the best for you.

Remember, here you are looking for a healthy lifestyle for the rest of your life, so it needs to be simple, flexible, and easy to follow, allowing you some "wiggle" room whenever you fancy something on the naughty list. If the food is high in calories or trans fats, it does not mean you can never eat it, it simply means that you need to adopt the moderation rule I mentioned earlier.

Many different types of food are ideal for menopause-aged women, since they contain micronutrients that can help overcome some of the negative effects of this time of life. For instance, magnesium is shown to help with bone mass and improve sleep; therefore, it is essential for menopausal women to include magnesium in their diet. This mineral is found in green leafy vegetables as well as in many fruits, nuts and seeds. In addition, vitamin C is essential for maintaining the health of your hair when you may be experiencing hair loss or thinning. This is one of the common menopausal symptoms and therefore it is advisable to consume foods rich in vitamin C, such as citrus fruits. Some women use vitamin C in the form of a supplement, but we will deal with this subject later.

Macronutrients are also known to provide your body with different benefits. For instance, carbohydrates will give you energy when you are feeling tired, and protein will help you feel fuller for longer, meaning you are less likely to give in to cravings or turn to unhealthy food options. Protein makes enzymes and hormones and is a building block of your muscle, skin and blood. Regarding fats, choosing to eat healthy types will help you lower the chances of heart disease and stroke. Healthy fats in your diet will rebuild your cells and stabilise your hormones.

You can see now how eating various foods, rather than relying on limited types, provides your body with everything it needs for healthy functioning and longevity.

Let's look in more detail at the types of foods you should be eating to help with your weight loss and other menopausal symptoms, and ensure that you follow a healthy diet in general.

Dairy Products

Dairy contains calcium, magnesium, phosphorus and vitamins K and D. These are all ideal vitamins to ensure bone health and strength. As you are probably aware, there is a chance of osteoporosis in later life if your bone density levels become too low due to a lack of oestrogen. This issue is particularly common with menopausal women. Consuming a substantial amount of dairy in the diet can help to prevent bone problems.

There is also a suggestion that dairy products may help to contribute towards a better night's sleep. This is because of the tryptophan found in dairy, which helps induce sleep. We have already talked about the fact that sleep can be affected during the menopausal period. A little later, I am going to talk in much more detail about sleep and how you can do your best to ensure that you are getting enough of it.

Healthy Fats, i.e. The Good Guys

When you hear the word "fat" you probably automatically think of the negative connotation, but the body needs a certain amount of fat in order to thrive.

There are good types of fat and there are bad ones too. Avoid the bad guys, such as trans fats, commonly found in processed meals, fried foods, and high-fat dairy products. Instead, focus on polyunsaturated fats, monounsaturated fats and omega 3 fatty acids.

Omega 3 fatty acids are commonly found in oily types of fish, such as salmon, anchovies and mackerel. If you are not a fish fan, you can also find them in some seeds, such as flax, hemp, chia, walnuts, pine nuts, and Brazil nuts in small amounts.

Of course, if you feel you are not getting enough Omega 3 through your food, then using a supplement, such as fish oil, might be a good option for you. It is essential to check out any supplements you consider taking with your doctor before you go ahead. It is common for supplements to interfere with any prescribed medication. For this reason, I strongly advise you to consult a medical practitioner about your intentions, to avoid any adverse effects of drug interactions that could damage your health.

Healthy types of fat not only help to regulate your weight and maintain satiety, reduce cravings for the harmful fats, but they may also reduce the severity of your hot flushes and night sweats. Again, this could help you get a better night's sleep if night sweats create a problem for you.

Primary sources of healthy fats include:

- Avocado

- Oily types of fish

- Olives

- Unsalted versions of nuts, cashew nuts, peanuts and almonds

- Oils made from seeds or plants, including extra-virgin olive oil, coconut oil, avocado oil, peanut oil, sesame oil, soybean oil, etc.

Eating healthy fat is necessary for your health. It provides your body with energy, protects you against heart disease, and helps your cells grow. Healthy fats can also support your weight loss by controlling your blood sugar levels and suppressing your appetite.

Wholegrains

The benefit of wholegrains for anyone trying to lose weight is that they are filling. This means you are less likely to snack on unhealthy options and are less likely to crave sugar and other unhealthy foods. Wholegrains are also high in fibre and vitamin B, which can benefit your overall health. Your body digests fibre more slowly than simple carbohydrates like starch and sugar, so the fibre from wholegrains keeps you feeling full for a more extended period.

We are all advised to eat wholegrains, regardless of age, because they offer many health benefits. When eaten as part of a balanced diet, they can protect against heart disease, diabetes and some types of cancer. The fact that wholegrains can keep you fuller for longer is a great way to deal with cravings and menopausal weight gain.

The types of foods to be on the lookout for include brown rice, rye, quinoa and barley.

Fresh Fruit and Vegetables

Everyone needs to get the right amount of fresh fruit and vegetables in their diet, regardless of gender or age. This used to be five a day, but then it went up to seven a day, and then there was some mention of 10. My advice? Do not bother trying to hit targets, just make sure that you pack your daily diet with plenty of fresh fruit and vegetables and you are good to go. There is no need to complicate matters further.

These products are brimming with a vast range of different vitamins and minerals and plenty of highly powerful antioxidants. These can keep you in optimum health and also keep your immune system strong. It has been shown that plenty of fresh fruit and vegetables, and fibre, may help postmenopausal women reduce the number of hot flushes and night sweats they experience.

If you want to know more about what you can do about those symptoms, I recommend you to have a look at my book *Free Yourself From Hot Flushes and Night Sweats: The Essential Guide to a Happy and Healthy Menopause*, which is available on Amazon.

Try and get the right amount of cruciferous vegetables into your diet too. This includes broccoli, cauliflower, kale, Brussels sprouts, cabbage and bok choy, to name a few, as well as colourful berries for powerful antioxidants.

Protein

Lean protein is vital for your overall health and well-being and is one of the main macronutrients that helps your body thrive. Consuming an adequate amount of protein ensures the healthy functioning of your body and contributes to bone health.

Remember, during the menopause, oestrogen declines, which is linked to decreased muscle mass, slowing down your metabolism and increasing the potential for lack of bone strength. Protein is required to protect against all of this.

The general guidelines are that menopausal women, over the age of 50 in particular, should eat 0.45-0.55 grams of lean protein per pound of their body weight. This is equal to 1-1.5 grams of lean protein per kilogram of their body weight. This averages out to around 20-25 grams of protein per meal if you weigh 10 stone or 63.5 kilograms.

For example, two eggs have around 26 grams of protein, and one steak has approximately 20 grams of protein.

You can also find a large quantity of protein in green leafy vegetables. This shows it is not so hard to meet your daily body needs and ensure you eat the right amount of protein.

To get a good amount of protein in your diet, you should look towards lean meat, fish, dairy products, eggs and legumes.

Water

Water is the most important nutrient that you can give to your body, whatever your age. Most of your body is made of water, and you keep losing it through sweating, breathing, urinating, etc. We even lose water while we sleep, and every milliliter of water needs to be replenished. Remember that the more you exercise, the more water you will need to drink. You also require more water if you live in a hot climate. I encourage you always to carry a water bottle. It will help you to stay hydrated.

Some of the benefits of drinking water include:

- Flushing out toxins

- Helping with digestion

- Regulating your body temperature

- Helping to prevent constipation

- Increasing energy

- Helping with weight loss

- Lubricating the joints

In my book, *Live Healthy on a Tight Schedule*, there is a section focusing on how to drink more water. Here are the key points of this section:

- Reports show that women should drink approximately 2.7 litres of water per day.

- Hydration can come from various sources, and some foods can be a good source of water.

- Foods that are very high in water content include various fruit and vegetables such as cucumbers, tomatoes, spinach, melon, oranges, broccoli, and berries.

- Consuming foods with a high water content not only helps you stay hydrated, but also provides you with fibre and various vitamins and minerals, all playing an essential role in keeping your body healthy.

- Drinking water needs to become a habit. Start by keeping a log of each time you drink water during the day, and estimate how much you have consumed.

Learn to appreciate water; it is the healthiest drink of them all.

Foods Which Contain Phytoestrogens

Certain types of food contain something called phytoestrogens. Now, anything with the word "oestrogen" in it should shout out to you as being useful for a menopausal woman, who suddenly finds herself lacking in this all-important hormone.

Phytoestrogens are found in some plants and act as a weak type of oestrogen which is in compound form. These are not the same as the hormone that declines in your body during the menopause, but they may help you deal with some particular symptoms, such as hot flushes. These types of foods are also healthy, so by packing these into your diet, you are also ensuring that you are on the right side of the health spectrum and you are doing your best to stay away from that pesky menopausal weight gain problem.

You may want to consider taking supplement called *Isoflavone* to reduce your menopausal symptoms. If this is the case, I suggest you ALWAYS check with your doctor if it safe for you to take it.

For naturally occurring phytoestrogens, look towards foods such as soy and red clover. The general advice is, if your diet is plant-based and is very rich in a variety of fruits, vegetables, legumes and some grains, then you are most likely consuming the necessary amounts of phytoestrogens through the food you eat.

So, now you know about the types of foods that are helpful for menopausal women, which will help you be healthy and avoid weight gain during this time in your life and in the future.

Now, let's look at which foods should you avoid?

This part is fairly easy and is the general advice that you would give anyone of any age if they have decided to become healthier and lose weight. However, certain foods may aggravate menopausal symptoms; you need to eliminate these for the time being to give you a more comfortable menopausal experience.

In general, you should avoid:

- **Foods containing added sugar** – Foods that may affect your blood sugar levels have been linked to an increase in hot flushes. A little later, we will talk about the role of blood sugar in weight gain, but for now, know that any foods that have added sugars are very unhealthy and not useful if you are struggling with hot flushes already. Sugar is linked to weight gain and increases the risks of diabetes, stroke and heart disease.

- *Processed carbohydrates* – Try and steer clear of baked goods (you can do it!) and white bread. These can increase your blood sugar levels and therefore contribute to hot flushes, while also being seriously bad for your waistline.

- *Alcohol* – Remember that watching what you drink is vital to controlling your weight. In addition to affecting your weight, alcohol prevents your body from absorbing vitamins and minerals. Therefore, alcoholic drinks are likely to have a significant impact on your overall health. Most alcoholic beverages are high in sugar, which will not help you battle your weight gain or control hot flushes. Remember, if you want a glass of wine or any other alcoholic beverage, do so in moderation. It is recommended that a menopausal woman should drink no more than one drink a day, which is equivalent to having seven drinks a week.

- **Spicy foods** – We are often told that eating spicy foods can be useful for weight loss because they help boost metabolism in some cases, but in terms of the menopause, the spice factor could make hot flushes worse.

- **Too much salt** – Excess amount of salt in food is not a healthy option for anyone. For a menopausal woman, it may lower your bone density over time, which could contribute to your chances of developing osteoporosis. Of course, the decrease in oestrogen also causes problems for your general health and your bones' health, but you can reduce this risk by reducing the amount of salt you eat.

Eating a healthy diet is not difficult in theory, but in practice, when you have got a million cravings coming your way and have never really tried to eat healthily before, it can be difficult. For the most part, you can find all the nutrients your body needs from the foods you eat, but in some cases, you may be tempted towards taking a supplement to improve your overall health or to manage some health conditions.

Before you take any type of supplement, be sure to consult your doctor. For the most part, many supplements are fine to take, but everyone's physiology is slightly different, therefore they will affect your health differently. I suggest you clear things with your doctor before beginning to use any supplement. This especially applies to you if you are taking any prescribed medication. Mixing supplements with certain medicines can be hazardous. Therefore, you must talk to your doctor about this.

Your doctor might recommends following supplements:

- Iron

- Evening primrose oil

- Potassium

- Magnesium

- Zinc

- Calcium

- Omega 3 fatty acids

- Vitamin A

- B vitamins, including B2, B6, B9 and B12

- Vitamin C

- Vitamin D

- Vitamin E

This is not an exhaustive list of the supplements your doctor may suggest you take. It will depend upon your health, diet, and current and past medical history.

Why Fad Diets do not Work

The last section was a lengthy one, but I hope that it crushed some myths about healthy eating and that you can now see that it is not particularly challenging to follow a healthy diet. You simply need to make healthy food choices. The more you do it, the more you will find yourself pulling away from unhealthy options, because you feel so great in yourself that you do not want to ruin it! You will also find that you can summon up the willpower to avoid giving in to cravings.

There are many ways you can meet your daily nutritional needs but following a fad diet is certainly not one of them. You should never go down the route of a fad diet. This type of diet is the one that does not support your health and it only focuses on weight loss. Fad diets do not strive to feed your body with quality foods such as organic fruit and vegetables or grass-fed meat for example, but instead they focus entirely on losing a few extra pounds in weight. Following a fad diet is not a sustainable way to live.

However, if you stick to a healthy, balanced diet, you will find that you are getting the right amount of nutrients, which is essential to your overall well-being.

I have mentioned the word "fad" a few times, and I want to explore this a little more before we move on.

I cannot stress enough that fad diets are not healthy. The companies and individuals behind these diets will tell you that they have discovered the quick route towards losing weight and that you will be in your bikini by the end of next week. They are lying! It is not possible to lose weight quickly and keep it off, not without severely damaging your health and making you miserable.

Any diet that involves counting points, advising you to stop consuming all kind of fat, permitting you to eat sugary and other unhealthy foods as long as you stick to your calorie allowance, or following theories that negatively impact your health, needs to go out the window. Keep it simple, and just choose healthy options over unhealthy ones. It is not rocket science. It works, but only if you commit to it.

Become food label savvy and understand that it is not good to eat it if the food is high in the wrong types of fat. Learn to grill, bake, or griddle your food rather than fry it and opt for healthy oils rather than unhealthy options. Snack on fruits and vegetables or nuts and seeds, rather than chocolate and ice cream, and know that there are hidden sugars in many drinks which claim to be "diet" or "zero calorie" versions. Water is always better and if you find it too bland, add a quick squeeze of fresh lemon or lime. Your body will benefit from the high level of vitamin C from these fruits.

Of course, the most important thing you should remember is that "M" word once again – moderation. Fad diets do not allow you to have anything you enjoy without ruining your hard work. If you crave a slice of pizza and follow a fad diet, you have zero chance of it being allowed. You will then have it anyway and feel bad that you have "ruined" your diet. This often leads to a binge session of all the foods you have missed so badly, which will make you feel much worse, telling yourself that you are a dietary failure and beat yourself up about it for weeks afterwards.

That is the damaging cycle of a fad diet.

I would like to remind you to visit bit.ly/menopause-healthy-recipes and download a free *Healthy Eating for Menopause – Recipe Book*. You will find simple and nutritious recipes that will support your health and weight loss goals.

When you eat healthily as much as possible, commit to moving your body more and enjoy your favourite foods in moderation, you are not restricting yourself to the point where you feel guilty for having a glass of wine or a few squares of chocolate. Life is too short to not feel the delicious melt of chocolate on your tongue or the zingy flavor of wine as it triggers your taste buds. Provided you do this in moderation, there is nothing to feel guilty about and no harm done. In some ways, it can even help you out, because it keeps your spirits up and ensures that you do not completely rebel against the new lifestyle you have chosen for yourself, which you intend to live for many years to come.

As you start to see results, you will feel so good about yourself that you will find it much easier to resist the cravings that your hormones might try and throw your way. This extra confidence will also help you to feel your best self as you go through the menopause. This is a time in life when many women feel less than their best, when they start to feel that they are getting older and perhaps missing out on the days of their youth. Of course, this is not the truth; menopause does not mean that anything is over, other than your periods – and for most women that is a good thing!

The more confident you are, the happier you are, the healthier you are, and the more able you are to deal with anything the menopause, or life in general, will throw at you. You will also find that it is much easier to lose weight because you are stuck on making healthy choices from this point onwards.

The Power of Journaling

Many women find it useful to keep a food journal. This works on many levels, but if you want to avoid making unhealthy food options, a food journal can show you where your trouble spots are and help put into place mechanisms to avoid falling foul of them in the future.

It is not unusual for your body to suddenly start to dislike a particular type of food or have a sensitivity or intolerance towards it, seemingly out of the blue. You might begin to notice stomach disturbances, bloating, or that you just do not feel your best after eating a specific ingredients. Keeping a food journal can help you identify this and then you can cut it out of your diet and see how that affects the way you feel.

Journaling is also an incredibly powerful tool for anyone trying to control their weight.

Invest in an attractive notebook and at the end of every day, write down what you ate for each meal, including drinks and snacks. Continue your journal for a couple of weeks in order to get a full picture of your eating habits. Be sure to note down anything you felt was out of the ordinary too. For instance, if you ate a cheese sandwich on white bread and you felt bloated straight afterwards, write it down. Then, look for other occurrences when you experienced bloating after eating white bread. If you notice it more than once, try changing white bread to wholemeal and see if you notice a difference.

Journaling is a great way to get a total overview of your dietary picture. You might think you are eating healthily, but it is only when you see what you consume over a day in black and white that you might realise just how unhealthy your diet is. Some people do not know how much sugar they eat until they reflect back on it, and others perhaps do not realise how much salt or alcohol they consume. A journal can give you this information and therefore put the control of your diet into your hands.

Journaling is useful for anyone trying to lose weight or improve their general health. It can help you to understand more about the foods you are craving. In your journal, be sure to write down when you have cravings and what types of foods you were desperate for.

You might find that at a specific point in the day, over several days, you are craving sugar. This can be resolved by changing your eating habits a little and perhaps eating some healthy snacks before that trouble hotspot time. You can then reassess for a bit longer and see if the craving subsides due to your direct actions.

A journal is also a useful way to identify whether you may need to start taking supplements. Before a doctor advises you to take some supplements, they will ask you about your general diet and may ask you to keep a journal for a couple of weeks. This will provide them with evidence of what you are lacking and what you might have too much of. Your journal will help them to identify what your body needs.

What Is Your Magic Number?

If you find that you need to lose weight, you must aim for a realistic weight for you. Just because a particular celebrity is a size zero, it does not mean that you need to be. Just because your friend is a size 10, it does not mean you should be the same size. We all have a magic number, a weight at which we feel comfortable, healthy and happy. Following advice from this book, you have a higher chance of reaching your healthy weight. You will be able to identify your magic number quite easily as you start to lose weight; it is the number at which your body simply settles. This is the weight that gives you confidence. It is the weight at which you do not put on weight easily, but you do not lose it either. It is your body's happy weight at which you are healthy and feel good in yourself.

When you reach that number, assuming it is a healthy one and that your BMI is within the healthy range, stay there and do not attempt to lose a little more in order to fit into a smaller dress size. Simply learn how to maintain it. Nobody is worth more or less just because they fit into a size 6, 8, 10, or anything over or above. As long as you are healthy and happy, that is really all that matters.

Before we move on from the subject of what a healthy diet should look like, I do need to mention one final thing on this topic. I have already touched upon the idea that during the menopause, decreased levels of oestrogen and progesterone can cause a blood sugar imbalance which can affect your weight gain and cause you mood swings, lack of sleep, depression or anxiety. Blood sugar imbalance is also known to lead to developing heart disease, obesity, type 2 diabetes, Alzheimer's disease and other life-threatening conditions. For this reason, you must control your blood sugar levels, which you can achieve comfortably through a healthy diet and lifestyle.

"Blood sugar balancing" is a simple way of managing your weight and keeping your body healthy. Let me briefly explain the basic principles of a blood sugar balancing diet, what it is and what you can do about it.

It is important to mention that if your diet is already reasonably healthy, you will not need to implement many changes, but if your diet is not very healthy, then pay attention to what I am about to say.

This is how blood sugar balancing works. After eating a meal, the food is broken down and turned into glucose (sugar), which then enters your bloodstream. Certain foods create more glucose than others, in which case your body produces more insulin. The role of insulin is to remove the sugar from the blood, but the downside is that insulin is a fat-storage hormone and causes weight gain. The key is to know which food spikes the blood sugar levels so that you can eat less of it. You also need to find out which foods are safe to eat so you can eat more of them and have a lean and healthy body.

As a general rule, this is how to keep your blood sugar balance stable throughout the day:

- Base your meals on protein and healthy fats. These two macronutrients are known to keep your blood sugar stable.

- Eat fibre-rich foods. This includes plenty of fruit and vegetables.

- Avoid foods with a high GI (glycemic index) rating and opt for foods with a low GI rating instead. Low GI foods include non-starchy vegetables such as lentils, green vegetables and green beans, while medium GI foods include oatmeal, sweet potatoes, peas and brown rice. Foods to avoid have a high GI and include white bread, white potatoes, white pasta, cakes, sweets, etc.

- Plan your meals ahead of time to ensure that you always have healthy foods at hand.

- Eat small meals more frequently throughout the day to avoid getting too hungry and then eating a large meal as this can spike your blood sugar levels.

- Take snacks out with you in your handbag or a car, so you are not tempted to opt for anything which could throw your blood sugar out of sync.

- Always eat breakfast. Make sure you avoid sugary cereals and start the day with a protein-based breakfast.

- Avoid sweetness or refined sugars and opt for natural sweeteners, such as honey or maple syrup, used in small amounts.

By keeping your blood sugar levels in check, you are contributing towards your overall health and well-being. By doing this, you are reducing risk factors that could lead to serious health concerns. It is important to mention that, in addition to health risks, blood sugar imbalance can cause irritability, fatigue, headaches or food cravings. Therefore, we turn to sugar-loaded carbohydrates, like pasta or bread, to gain energy to get on with our day.

My final advice in this chapter is to assess your weight and ask yourself the following question: do you need to lose weight because your current weight puts your health at risk? If so, make changes to your diet and lifestyle as described in this book to reduce your weight in a slow and steady manner. Fad diets might promise you a massive weight loss within a short period of time, but such an approach is totally unsustainable over the long term.

It is important to ensure that you are working towards realistic targets and you are not trying to aim towards something that is completely out of reach, unsustainable or unhealthy. It is fine to be curvy, provided you are healthy on the inside. Equally, it is fine to be slim or skinny as long as you are healthy on the inside. There is no "one size fits all" answer here; it entirely depends on your body type, genetics, health, and ideal aim. Just make sure that whatever that aim is, it is realistic and achievable for you.

My advice is to keep your lifestyle healthy even after you have lost the weight. By doing this, you will be able to manage any possible weight gain as a result of the menopause.

Key Points

We have covered a lot of ground in this chapter. However, everything I have shared with you is super-useful and super-relevant to your health in general. There is never a negative side to being healthy; you really are what you eat and that means you need to be careful of what you are putting into your body if you want to look and feel your best.

We also know that the hormonal effects of the menopause have a nasty habit of causing weight gain if you are not clued up beforehand on what may happen. Far too many women are unaware that weight gain is a possible side effect of the menopause, and then they are shocked when they get on the scales or notice that their clothes are becoming tighter.

It is much harder to lose weight as you get older, simply because your metabolism is not as fast as it used to be. Keeping and maintaining a healthy weight during this time will make life easier for you, keep your confidence levels up and help you handle the effects of the menopause more comfortably and positively.

Here are the main points to take from this chapter:

- Health and well-being should be at the forefront of your mind at all times, ensuring that you battle any potential menopause weight gain before it begins.

- Vitamins and minerals that are essential to a menopausal woman include magnesium, calcium, B vitamins, etc. They can be consumed through a healthy diet or by taking supplements.

- Eating a balanced diet will ensure you get a range of macronutrients and micronutrients.

- Fad diets are to be avoided. Anything that is causing you to restrict your intake to significant levels is not necessary (unless a medical practitioner suggests it due to health reasons) and is likely to cause you to rebel against just how restrictive the diet is. Avoid at all costs is my advice!

- Moderation is key! You can have a little of what you fancy, even if it falls within the "bad for you" category, provided you pull back on other days and only have it occasionally and in a small amount.

- Changes to your diet have to be a lifestyle change and not something you only follow for a few weeks; if you do that, any weight you lose will return afterwards.

- You always need to speak to a qualified person to get the best advice if you feel that you are not getting the optimal range of vitamins and minerals in your diet and also if you are looking at getting supplements.

- During the menopause, hormonal imbalance can cause blood sugar to become unstable. Therefore, you need to make sure that you consume a healthy diet, which includes eating little and often and avoiding any foods which are known to spike your blood sugar quickly, such as baked goods and high GI rated foods.

- If you need to lose weight, make sure that you are choosing a weight that is realistic for you and is not going to push you to painful and unhealthy limits.

Chapter 5

The Vital Role of Exercise

At any stage of life, you need to keep your body healthy and strong. This is especially important for women going through the menopause when all manner of changes occur. It is easy to put exercise to one side, assuming that we do not have time, or it is simply too hard. There are countless ways you can incorporate a little more movement into your day and therefore obtain the significant benefits of exercise.

You do not have to join the gym, or hire a personal trainer, or sweat it out every single day to become a healthier person; you simply need to eat healthily, ensure you are getting a range of vitamins and minerals, and move your body more. That is what exercise is, in its most simplistic form — it is moving your body more.

At this stage in your life, exercise is vital.

In this chapter, I will talk about the benefits of exercising and give you some ideas and inspiration regarding the best types of exercise for menopausal women. You will also learn how physical activity can easily fit into a healthy lifestyle.

Exercise does not have to be torture. It can be fun! Look at Zumba classes for a start — sure, they make you sweat, but they are great fun and help you make new friends too. My idea of fun is to go swimming and play tennis. I have a few more hobbies that I enjoy doing, but these two are very much part of my life and have been for years.

There is no downside when it comes to exercising regularly, but like everything else, you should not overdo it either. That is also something I want to talk about. You need to find the sweet spot — the amount of exercise that is healthy for you, giving you benefits and not making you feel exhausted and causing more problems than it is worth. What I am trying to say here is that pushing your body too hard through exercise might not bring the desired benefits, but instead it will be causing some damage.

The body of a menopausal woman needs the right type of exercise as much as it needs rest; otherwise, the combination of too much exercise and going through hormonal changes, are likely to cause stress and push your body to the limit. This might lead to adrenal fatigue, which is why finding the right exercise during this stage of your life is crucial.

The most common symptoms of adrenal fatigue include anxiety, having difficulties sleeping, craving sugary and salty foods, experiencing a lack of energy and reduced tolerance to stress.

We know that during the menopause weight gain is probable. We also know that menopausal women are at high risk of developing visceral fat around the middle and around the abdominal area. It has been proven that those are the hardest types of fat to lose. We also know that regular exercise will not only help prevent weight gain but also help lose the excess weight that you already carry. In addition, taking regular exercise that is right for your body will decrease the likelihood of having your weight creep back on after the menopause is over.

Exercise Is Key for the Mind, Body and Soul

There is no such thing as a healthy lifestyle without exercise. However, the exercise you choose to do has to be enjoyable for you and tweaked in a way that cannot cause you any harm. For instance, if you have a bad back already, you need to alter how you do exercises to avoid putting extra strain on your back and avoid causing any other injuries as a result. If you are not sure how to do this, have a chat with a personal trainer at your gym, or talk to your doctor or physiotherapist. They will be able to give you advice on the best types of exercise for you and how you can modify mainstream exercises to suit your situation and any pre-existing injuries or conditions you have.

It is recommended that adults get around 150 minutes of moderate exercise every week, at least. Alternatively, you can get 75 minutes per week of higher intensity exercise. This type of activity requires you to move your body faster, get your heart rate up and sweat a little. This does not have to be every single day. You can focus on the moderate or the intense exercises or mix them together in a full workout that you do less often. It is up to you how you want to approach your exercise regime.

To make it a long-term plan, you need to fit your workout into your lifestyle and routine. It is better and more beneficial to exercise a little every day, rather than doing a full-on workout once or twice a week. If you spread it out over the week, you are getting continual benefits.

A little later, I will talk about the types of exercise you might like to try and why they are useful for menopausal women, but for now let me give you some idea of what moderate and intense exercise look like.

With moderate exercise, you will be able to talk while you are doing it, but not hold a full conversation. You can say a few words if you need to and will not be out of breath as a result.

Intense exercise means that you need to stop to breathe in between words because it is not possible to speak while you are doing it. These exercise types need to be aerobic, i.e. you are getting your heart rate up and you are sweating a little. It could mean walking fast, jogging, running on the spot, etc. You should also do some form of strengthening exercise ideally twice per week. This will ensure that you are maintaining your muscle mass, which reduces the chances of putting on weight, and strengthening your bones at the same time.

You might be wondering what strengthening exercises look like? The most basic strengthening exercises include push-ups, sit-ups and arm lifts with small hand weights.

It is important to mention that moderate and intense types of exercises are both equally beneficial for menopausal women.

You might be surprised to hear that exercise is not just beneficial for your body, but it is also a fantastic way to keep your spirits up. If you think back to our chapter on stress management, exercise was one of the main ways to keep stress and low mood at bay.

When you exercise, your body releases several feel-good chemicals such as endorphins and dopamine, known to make you feel a natural high. This is partly to help your body to handle the exercise you are doing, but it has the beneficial side effect of boosting your mood at the same time. The more regularly you exercise, the more often you experience this natural high and the better you feel in general.

Of course, low mood and anxiety are common symptoms for menopausal women, so exercising regularly can help you handle these in addition to keeping menopausal weight gain down and strengthening the body.

Be determined to exercise regularly over the next couple of weeks and think honestly about how you feel afterwards. Sure, you might have to wash your sweaty clothes a little more often, but that is a small price to pay when you consider the feel-good factor you will experience as a result!

So, what are the actual benefits of exercise in detail?

Weight Control

It goes without saying that if you eat a healthy diet and exercise regularly, you will likely lose excess weight and keep your weight down. Exercise is a vital weapon in the battle against obesity, but you need to be sure that you are eating healthily alongside it. No amount of exercise will allow you to burn off the calories you consumed if you eat pizza, cakes and burgers every day.

Heart Disease Risk Reduction

The risk of developing heart disease and associated complications are often present as we become a little older, especially as we enter the menopause.

Decreased levels of oestrogen during the menopause can cause LDL cholesterol to rise. That is a "bad type" of cholesterol that is harmful to us and can lead to heart attack and stroke. Exercise plays a vital role in reducing that risk.

When you exercise, you increase the amount of oxygen in your body and improve circulation. Your circulatory system carries oxygen, nutrients and hormones to cells and helps your body to remove carbon dioxide. This plays a part in reducing the risk of heart disease and it also increases the possibility of keeping your body healthy.

Regular exercise can lower your cholesterol and blood pressure. It can also reduce your blood sugar levels, which lowers your risk of becoming obese and developing diabetes. However, this relies upon you eating a healthy diet alongside the exercise.

In addition to these benefits, regular exercise is also believed to reduce your risk of developing certain types of cancer, including breast, uterine, lung and colon cancer.

Mood Improvement and Anxiety Reduction

As I have already mentioned, it is not unusual for a woman to feel down, stressed or anxious during the menopause. It is a result of hormonal changes, the overall stress of what is happening within her body, and could also be from not sleeping well.

Exercise can help you manage this and lift your mood. You will also feel more positive about the changes that are happening inside your body and find it easier to cope with the process as a result.

As I already mentioned, when you exercise, your body releases feel-good chemicals. You will smile more and feel happier, and the effects will last long after you have taken your last movement and sat down for a break. You will feel relaxed and have a sense of achievement too. This all helps you deal with the menopausal symptoms and keep your mood and general feel-good factor up. After endorphins are released inside your body, you will be in a better mood and have more energy as a result. This happy feeling can last for hours after exercising.

Serotonin is another happy hormone that can be affected by exercise. Studies show that cardio exercises are great for boosting serotonin levels, which not only positively affect your mood, but make a difference to your sleep, sexual desire, memory, appetite and digestion.

Mind Strengthening

Brain function is a "use it or lose it" kind of deal and it is essential to regularly challenge yourself to keep your cognitive function up to optimal levels. This applies to any age, but when you are going through the menopause, the hormonal rollercoaster and brain fog you experience make it difficult to concentrate or focus.

When we exercise, the body drives oxygen and blood to the brain, keeping the mind sharper. During exercise, the body releases proteins and endorphins. These not only make us feel good and help strengthen and improve brain function, but they also improve blood circulation, which benefits the brain and improves its sharpness.

Bones and Muscles Strengthening

I have mentioned that women lose muscle mass during the menopause, leading to possible weight gain and weakening of the bones and developing osteoporosis in later life.

Regular exercise can reduce this risk by keeping your muscles and bones as strong as possible. As a result, your bone density levels will be higher, and your muscle mass will remain optimal, which will help you control weight gain.

Sleep Improvement

While it is not a good idea to exercise right before you sleep (endorphins will flood your body making you feel too active to fall asleep), regular exercise during the day can help you relax and, therefore, sleep better.

Ensuring you get enough exercise throughout the week while checking your sleeping routine (more on that shortly) can allow you to fall asleep much faster than otherwise, avoiding those annoying nights of broken sleep. All of this means you will be more energised, focused and able to handle the challenges that the menopause may bring. From a weight management point of view, sleep is also vital.

Libido Improvement

Due to the lowered oestrogen and progesterone levels you will experience during menopause, you may find that your desire for sexual intercourse is a lot lower than usual. It might be up and down and all over the place, but you will find that these levels are improved by exercising regularly. This is all down to increased circulation and those feel-good chemicals. Whether this is a plus point for you or not is a personal matter, but it can certainly be a valuable benefit for many.

As you can see, exercise has a range of benefits, not only for the body but for the mind and soul too. You will feel better, be more relaxed, look better, be stronger, and you will be able to manage your weight much more effectively. Again, it is vital that you combine exercise with a healthy diet – one does not work without the other, so make sure that you are ticking both boxes to receive the significant benefits on offer.

Exercise is one thing you can do for free that will make many of your menopausal symptoms more manageable. As you will see in the next sections, you can add extra enjoyment to it by working with a friend or merely finding an activity that interests you.

Finding Your Perfect Exercise

There are countless types of exercise you can try, and you can stick to the kind of exercise you like, or you can mix things up occasionally. You do not need to do anything you do not enjoy, so if you are not a fan of going to the gym, you do not have to go. If you are not a fan of getting into a swimsuit, no-one is forcing you to. If you want, you can download an app on your smartphone and try yoga in the comfort of your home. There are no rules to this; you simply go with what feels right to you.

There is a myth that exercising has to be hard work, you have to sweat, wear rather unflattering lycra, and spend a small fortune on a gym membership, which you must use several times per week without fail. None of this is true.

Yes, exercise is hard work, but it can be done in a way that makes it feel less so, by doing something you enjoy. Nobody is pushing you to join a gym if you are not keen or if you simply cannot afford the rather costly membership fees.

If you would rather exercise in the comfort of your own home than in public, I recommend you read my book, *Get Fit and Healthy in Your Own Home in 20 Minutes or Less*. In this book, you will find a daily exercise plan with plenty of home workouts and simple meal ideas to help you lose weight and get the body you want. The exercises I shared in this book are easy to follow and suitable for the needs of menopausal women. The book is available on Amazon.

Living healthily does not need to be expensive or time consuming, but one thing that a healthy lifestyle needs from you is your commitment. You need to commit to eating nutritious foods and moving your body as often as you can. You must also remember to include other aspects of self-care. They are equally important.

There are countless ways you can weave exercise into your routine and many small things you can do every day to get your body moving more. These are the types of things we will talk about in this section.

The bottom line is that even small changes to your daily routine can make a difference. Here are a few suggestions:

- Walk to work rather than use the car.

- Get off the bus a couple of stops earlier than you usually would and walk the rest of the way.

- Take the steps instead of the lift.

- Go for a walk on your lunch break, rather than sit at your desk.

- When you talk to friends on the phone, walk around the room as you do it, rather than sit on the sofa.

- Washing your car is another excellent way of getting a full-body exercise that works with most of your muscle groups, particularly your upper body: chest, shoulders and arms.

- Gardening is another great way of implementing movement in your everyday life.

I have just shown you that even if you never place a foot inside the gym, there are many things you can do to keep your body in shape.

Of course, we know that it is important you also have to do some formal exercise, i.e. an activity which gets your blood flowing and your heart rate up. While going through the menopause, many women feel unsure of their health because so many changes are occurring at the same time. Doing regular exercise can help any person improve their health, and it is very common for the exercise to alleviate some of the symptoms associated with the menopause. Trust me on this!

In this book, I am not promoting any specific activity, as it is up to you which one you go for, but the following are a few suggestions which may be useful for menopausal women in particular.

I would like to remind you that before you start with any type of exercise, it is important to have a quick chat with your doctor if you have any pre-existing conditions or any specific limitations in your mobility, e.g. a regularly sore back or arthritis.

Doing exercises that are not suitable for your condition could be quite damaging. Make sure that you always look after your body.

- *Join an exercise class* – By joining a class, you gain an extra boost in confidence because it is a social activity at the same time. If you opt for a class for your particular age group, you will probably feel more comfortable. How about Zumba or even belly dancing? Go for something you have always wanted to try but never felt able to and see how great it feels when you master a new activity.

- *Brisk walking outdoors* – Heading outdoors means you are getting a boost of vitamin D and serotonin from the sun, but always remember to practice sun safety. Brisk walking is also a great way to get some aerobic exercise, working your lungs and getting your heart rate up. This helps to burn calories and therefore manage your weight. Of course, aerobic exercise also helps to protect against heart disease. If you want to add a touch of strength training, you simply need to carry a small set of hand weights as you are walking.

- **Hiking** – If you love the outdoors and you are relatively fit, why not put on your walking boots and head out into the countryside, to the coast, or the nearest mountain? This is a great way to get all the benefits of being outside while enjoying aerobic exercise. Of course, be sure to check the weather and always listen to your body.

- **Jogging** – If you have never tried jogging before, start slow and build up as you go. Head to the nearest park and enjoy the scenery while grabbing some much-needed aerobic exercise. This can also help build up strength in the legs, contributing to muscle and bone health. It is perfectly fine to do spurts of just 10 minutes, which should be achievable after a few introductory sessions if you have never done jogging before. All you need to do is do three sets and rest between intervals to take you up to your half an hour of aerobic exercise a day.

- **Swimming** – Swimming is the ideal combination of strength training and aerobic exercise because of the water-resistance. We know that strength training is vital for menopausal women to prevent bone density loss and preserves as much muscle mass as possible. Swimming is probably one of the most gentle ways to achieve this type of exercise.

Of course, being in the water is also very calming and relaxing, which could help you deal with any anxiety you may be experiencing and help you get a good night's sleep.

- **Join the gym** – If you want to try joining the gym, then go for it. Most gyms have introductory sessions and you have the services of a personal trainer or instructor to hand if you want further advice. This can be useful if you have never really used gym equipment before and if you have any conditions that mean specific exercises need to be adapted for your needs. You also get the option of using machinery to help with strength training while combining it with your aerobic needs.

- **Yoga and Pilates** – Yoga and Pilates are both ideal activities for menopausal women because they help with flexibility and strength while also building muscle mass. Of course, they are both very relaxing activities, especially yoga, which teaches you to focus on breathing to overcome difficulties and help you move into various positions. There is a suggestion that yoga can help with sleep issues by relaxing you and easing sore muscles that may be holding tension. If you have any problems with mobility, it is crucial to speak to the instructor before the class begins, and they will show you how to alter the poses for your particular needs.

- ***Join the club*** – Joining your local tennis or golf club is a great idea. There are many sports you can start playing at any age. I named two of them as an example, but nothing stops you from joining any club and starting a new sport. It does not matter if your age is 40-plus or 50-plus; learning a sport you have never played before will raise your confidence and help you develop new skills. It will also build your fitness level, improve your health and maintain a healthy weight. Of course, you also get to meet new people there.

This is not an exhaustive list of sporting activities you can try, but those mentioned are specifically useful for women of a menopausal age because they help to reduce many menopausal symptoms and offer a combination of aerobic and strength exercises.

Do not Overdo It!

There is a common way of thinking that you need to be "all in" when it comes to exercise, but that is not the case. As long as you are doing as much as you can do comfortably and you are doing it regularly, that is enough. You do not have to push yourself to extremes. You are only going to end up injured or develop aches and pains if you do.

It is vital that before you start any exercise session, regardless of what it is, you do some stretches to warm your muscles up. If you go into your exercise cold, you might end up with a pulled muscle and possibly worse. Your body is already under enough stress at this time of your life, so do not add extra fuel to the fire by attempting to exercise without warming up. Warm-up exercises are designed to warm your muscles and prepare your body for exercise. Stretches are easy enough to do and you should not overextend to the point of pain either — simply feeling a gentle pull is all you need.

You should also stretch after you have exercised; this is called a cool down. Stretching exercises relax and restore your muscles after the workout. This helps your muscles remain flexible, which can be a problem during menopause. If you do not do this, your muscles will feel tight and painful the next day, and perhaps you will struggle to move.

Cooling down helps protect the wide range of motion in all major muscle groups and ensures that your joints remain flexible and healthy. Remember, these are areas of the body that can deteriorate as you age. While I am not suggesting that you are ready to start drawing your pension payments, you do need to start protecting your body for your later years — the ideal time is now.

Stretching also helps with stability, which will help you when you get much older and may be more susceptible to falls. Being flexible and supple is never a bad thing, and you will feel fitter and healthier for far longer by following this advice.

In the book I mentioned earlier, *Get Fit and Healthy in Your Own Home in 20 Minutes or Less*, you will find plenty of warm-up and stretching exercises. Both types of exercises can prevent your body from strain and injuries and keep it in good form.

It goes without saying that you should stay hydrated during your exercise sessions and make sure that you drink plenty of water. If you feel lightheaded or you are sweating excessively, sit down and take a break. You should not feel this way during regular exercise. Do not push yourself to your extreme limits; you simply need to move your body more and get your heart rate up a little. That is all! Anything more than that and you are putting yourself at risk of injury and illness — and that is not what we are aiming for.

Remember, your body is under enough stress as it is; you simply need to take some of the strain away by helping it out with some healthy exercise along with a healthy diet. By trying to do too much, especially if you have never really had an exercise routine before, you are going to end up feeling terrible afterwards and probably be put off exercising ever again.

Moving your body and exercising regularly is the key to your success — remember this! Overdoing it once in a while or pushing yourself to the extreme levels on a daily basis is not what your body needs.

The key is to find an exercise that you enjoy, dedicate time to it and make it a priority. If exercising feels like a chore and you are dreading exercise time or simply do not enjoy what you are doing, you have likely chosen the wrong type of exercise. I suggest you think again and look at different options.

Exercising is something you need to feel happy and comfortable doing over the long term. Doing the right type of exercise is crucial. When you do something you love, you will feel much happier and more positive. Feeling this way will motivate you to create a habit of exercising regularly.

Finding an Exercise Buddy

Many women find exercising alone to be a lonely business. Of course, not everyone feels this way, but if you do, why not find an exercise buddy and make your active time a social time too? This can be ideal for banishing stress, and if you exercise with another woman your age, you can share your experiences of the menopause with each other. You will be able to understand each other's struggles.

Exercising with other people is the reason why many women choose to attend an exercise class. If you look around your local area, I am sure you will find classes catering only for women over the age of 40 or 50. This could help you meet other women who are going through this time in life and give you support. Besides, other people can motivate us when we are feeling tired, uninspired or lazy.

Making exercise fun is not as difficult as you think. Yes, your muscles might burn and you are going to be a little out of breath, but as I mentioned before, if you choose an exercise that you enjoy, you will not notice the downsides. You are also strengthening your body and helping to maintain your weight. That pesky menopausal weight gain issue is something which most women deal with, but exercise, along with a healthy diet, will help you to master the problem with far greater ease than otherwise.

So, how else can you make exercise fun?

- **Download a tracking app** – Many women like to use pedometers, but how about downloading an app that measures how many steps you are taking throughout the day. There are apps that could help you compete against family or friends, measuring who makes a higher number of steps per day. That is a great motivator and an excellent way to make exercise fun and competitive, rather than something you simply have to do.

- **Make sure you go outside** – Again, we have talked about this, but it is vital to put it in this section too. Exercising outdoors makes it more fun because of the fresh air and the new environment, and it is excellent for your mood. Natural light and fresh air can boost your immune system and strengthen your mental health, which will benefit you while navigating the menopausal journey.

- **Exercise at different times of the day** – Mix your routine up and exercise at different times. Doing this can stop your exercise routine from becoming tedious and help you discover your favourite time of the day to exercise. You might be doing it in the morning simply because you think that is the best time, but if you do not try a few different options, how will you really know? When you find your favourite time to exercise, then stick to it and put it in your diary.

- **_Keep an exercise journal_** – When you choose a new exercise or activity, it is a good idea to keep a journal and write down your experiences. Journaling will help you understand how you feel about it and whether it is the right one for you.

Should you weigh yourself every day?

I do not recommend you weigh yourself too often. Our weight fluctuates naturally throughout the day and even across the week, so weighing yourself every day is going to give you unhelpful information. If you do not see the results you want, it could damage your confidence.

Weigh yourself once a week and always do it at the same time, simply so you know whether your weight is going up, down, or it is staying the same. Whatever the number you see on the scale, do not allow it to upset you. Weight loss is a journey like any other — sometimes smooth and sometimes rough. The changes you are going to make to your lifestyle will be far-reaching, and that is something you need to have faith in at this point.

Weighing yourself daily could be disempowering if you do not see a massive difference in numbers, but do not panic; it is better to measure your progress according to how you feel. This is the advice I always give to my clients.

Instead of focusing on the number on the scale, I suggest you pay attention to the following:

- Do you have more energy?

- Are you sleeping better?

- What are your menopausal symptoms like at this point?

The weight loss will come as you continue with your healthy lifestyle via a balanced diet and regular exercise. When you are preparing healthy foods or sweating on the gym floor or in the park, think about all the health benefits you are achieving by doing this, rather than how much you weigh.

The way we feel is much more important. Besides, fat loss sometimes comes before weight loss. This means that your clothes will fit you better, your posture will improve, but the scale will show the opposite. This is the harsh reality of weight loss. That is why you should not focus solely on the number on the scale but also on the positive side effects of your healthy lifestyle and healthy attitude towards your body.

I previously mentioned an exercise journal and also talked about a food journal that could help you find out how different foods make you feel. You can combine these journals to look at patterns and spot trends.

When you do weigh yourself, jot these numbers down and look for the downward trend. If you notice the numbers going up a little, you can search through your journal for any clues as to why this is the case.

Some of my clients tell me that they are finding it more challenging to lose weight, and sometimes they even notice their weight went up following a period of poor sleep.

The lack of sleep contributes to their low energy levels, so they exercise less. Poor sleep is also associated with consuming more sugary loaded foods and simple carbohydrates. Unhealthy food choices are often linked to increased levels of ghrelins — a hunger hormone caused by a lack of sleep.

I already talked about the importance of good sleep, and I highly recommend focusing on it as a main priority. Without proper rest, you might find it very hard to have a healthy body and a healthy mind. We will talk more about this topic in the next chapter.

Remember, you are aiming for a new lifestyle for the rest of your years, not for just a few weeks or months.

Key Points

In this chapter, I have talked at length about exercise. You might not have initially loved the idea of being more active, but I hope I have inspired you to think about taking up a new activity or perhaps re-starting one which you may have done in the past.

I want you to remember these key points from this section:

- Exercise is vital for overall health and well-being and is an essential tool in managing your weight.

- Regular exercise has a range of benefits, including weight management, reducing the risk of heart disease, promoting better sleep and strengthening bones and muscles. All of these benefits are vital for a menopausal woman.

- It is no good exercising if you are not eating in the right way. Regular exercise and healthy eating need to be close partners if you want to gain the greatest benefits.

- Find an exercise activity that you enjoy — exercise should not be a chore; it should be something you like to do and something which makes you feel good.

- Remember to have a combination of aerobic and strength training exercises and always warm up and cool down too.

- If you are starting a new exercise activity and have a condition or pre-existing injury, consult your doctor to find out how you can adapt the exercise to suit your needs.

Chapter 6

Sleep Your Way to Weight Loss?

Who does not love a good night's sleep?

That wonderful feeling when you wake up in the morning, look at your alarm clock and realise that you have another three hours before you have to get up. Ahh, bliss! You turn back over, snuggling into your duvet and allow yourself to drift back off.

Sleep is not just an enjoyable thing; it is also vital for having a healthy body and mind. We need sleep for a very good reason. Unfortunately, during the menopause, many women find their sleep pattern disturbed and some may even struggle with insomnia.

Why is this?

Again, it is attributed to hormones and how they affect the human body. I have already mentioned that as you enter the menopause, the two primary hormones, progesterone and oestrogen, start to dwindle. The problem is, progesterone is the hormone that helps you fall asleep. So, when it is in low supply, you begin to struggle with getting a good night's sleep. You might find it hard to fall asleep, or wake up several times during the night, thereby leaving you feeling exhausted the next day.

Night sweats can also be a problem when you are trying to sleep. When this happens, your body is experiencing a quick hit of adrenaline, and again, that is not conducive to relaxation and sleep. It is part and parcel of the fight or flight stress response I talked about earlier. Experiencing night sweats several times per night and over a long period of time (with some women it lasts for months or even years), as we already know, can become dangerous in terms of a prolonged stress response and a lack of sleep.

You might also struggle with sleep as a result of anxiety. It is normal to feel worried and confused during any changes in your life, and the menopause is a pretty big one. In this case, you may find yourself overthinking when you are at your quietest moment, meaning that you struggle to go to sleep or have difficult dreams.

Of course, it is crucial that you do your best to have as good a night's sleep as possible. We all need to rest. During sleep, the body focuses on regeneration, healing, and replenishing energy for the next day. In addition, your body is changing, which means you need to rest to allow it to complete the process it needs to go through.

In this chapter, I am going to talk in more detail about how you can make changes in your lifestyle to help you find the sweet spot for sleep.

The Undeniable Connection Between Sleep and Weight

Sleep, sleep, sleep... It is essential not only for managing your weight loss but also for maintaining your overall health and well-being. Many health conditions can be improved simply by getting better rest on a more consistent basis. If you are not sleeping well, your immune system will be affected, and you will be more at risk of developing some life-threatening conditions. Also, you are more likely to put weight on. Have you noticed this?

Sleep was one of the few things that our parents made sure we had enough of when we were babies, but we all tend to abandon it when we reach our teenage years. This is quite possibly one of the first good habits we give up on in life.

Establishing a consistent sleep schedule will help you get a better sleep quality every night, helping you be the best version of yourself each day.

One of the best analogies I have ever heard compared sporadic bedtimes to jet lag. Whether you lose 3 hours or 13 hours to a flight, you know your entire body simply feels off when you jump through time zones. Every time you go to sleep one hour later than usual, your natural rhythm is disrupted.

We have become so used to feeling like this that now we assume it is perfectly normal. In fact, sleeping more hours and having a better quality of sleep will provide us with better health and more energy.

Numerous studies show the positive effects of sleep on our well-being and many found a strong correlation between lack of sleep and weight gain.

In 2013, a study conducted by the University of Colorado investigated how sleep affects eating and gaining weight. The results concluded that sleeping just five hours a night over only one week leads to putting on around two pounds in weight. According to these findings, it would mean that if you sleep that long every night over a month, that is eight pounds in weight, gained simply by not sleeping enough.

The study showed that your hunger signals simply do not shut off when you do not get enough sleep, leading you to consume extra 500-plus calories in one day.

The average adult is supposed to get between seven to eight hours of sleep every night. Of course, most people do not hit that spot every night, but on average, that is the best duration we should aim for. Anything less than that will have an impact on our health, energy, or mood.

The problem of weight gain comes when there is a lack of sleep, i.e. you are sleep deprived. You are classed as being sleep deprived when you get less sleep than the seven to eight hours recommended, even for just a few nights, and you are experiencing the following symptoms:

- Feeling very sleepy during the daytime

- Excessive yawning

- Feeling moody or snappy

- Forgetting things easily

- General fatigue

- Low mood

- Not being able to concentrate or handle anything new which is presented to you, i.e. difficulty taking on new ideas or concepts

Some of those symptoms overlap with the menopause, making it challenging to figure out the real problem. However, if you are finding it hard to fall asleep, you wake up often, you do not want to get out of bed in the mornings and you are struggling with tiredness throughout the day, I advise you to change your routine and do your best to address your sleep problem.

When you are sleep deprived, some hormonal imbalances occur within your body. I am talking here about hunger and satiation hormones, ghrelin and leptin. When you are not getting enough sleep, the levels of these two hormones are affected. Therefore, you feel hungrier, and your body does not notice when you are full quite as easily.

Here is a brief explanation of how they work and how they are affected by your sleep.

Ghrelin is the hormone that is responsible for telling your brain when you need to eat. And leptin tells your brain when you are full. In other words, ghrelin increases the appetite, while leptin decreases the appetite.

During a good night's sleep, the ghrelin levels will decrease, and leptin levels will increase. If you did not have a good night's sleep, your hormones would be affected, and your ghrelin levels will be increased, which means that you will be eating more. On the other hand, your leptin levels will be decreased. Therefore, your body will not know when it is full, and as a result, you will feel hungrier and eat more before feeling full up.

This is the perfect storm for weight gain because it leads you to make unhealthy food choices and overeat. As I have mentioned before, you are more likely to be tempted towards foods which are high in unhealthy fat and sugar and of course, these are the types of foods that will make you pile on the pounds. The fact that you are sleep deprived means that you cannot make clear and sensible decisions, so you are more likely to overeat too. Many studies have shown this, and unfortunately, I experienced it myself.

We also know that getting older affects your muscle mass, and from the age of 30 we begin to lose muscle mass by 3-

8% per decade. After the age of 60, the rate we lose muscle mass is increased. But do not worry! It has been proven that leading a healthy lifestyle can help us build muscle at any age. Including good nutrition and regular exercise in your daily routine you can reverse the process and slow down muscle mass decrease.

Sleep is another essential factor that is crucial for maintaining muscle mass. When you are not getting enough sleep, the muscle mass is at a critical level. The lower your muscle mass, the more difficult it will be to maintain your healthy weight.

As you can see, sleep is vital and not just something we like to do at night when we are feeling a little tired and want to forget about the day's worries. The good news is that if you are having problems with sleep during your menopausal period, there are many things you can do to change your lifestyle and give yourself a better chance of having a full seven to eight hours of sleep every night.

10 Ways to Get a Better Night's Sleep

In this section, I am going to talk to you about changing your routine to increase your chances of getting a good night's sleep regularly. You might not struggle with sleep every night, but most women going through the menopause have disturbances at some point, either every few nights or for a prolonged period.

Establishing a routine prepares the body and brain for falling asleep faster; therefore, I suggest you explore the ideas I am going to share with you. These methods are worth looking into even if some of the problems I mentioned do not apply to you.

Go to Bed and Wake up At the Same Time Every Day

You might be tempted to have a lie-in at the weekend, but I would not suggest it. It is a better idea to maintain a routine when it comes to sleep. That means going to bed at the same time every day and setting your alarm for the same time every day too. Sure, it is not going to hurt if you have a special function to attend and go to bed a little later one night, but anything more than that will start sending you into sleep deprivation territory.

Going to bed at the same time, and getting the same amount of sleep every night will make you feel remarkably more alert and energised, and probably help you get slimmer and healthier too. Your body clock is consistent by maintaining a routine, and your hormones will remain in sync far more easily.

Balanced hormones support your physical, mental, and emotional state, and allow you to thrive.

Avoid Anything Too Stimulating Before Bed

It is not a good idea to watch TV till late at night, listen to fast or loud music, or spend hours on your laptop or tablet before you sleep. Instead, listen to chilled out music, read a book and have a warm bath before bedtime. These activities will put you in a more relaxed frame of mind and help you to wind down. Anything too stimulating will just make it harder for you to switch off and will keep you awake.

Rigorous exercising just before bedtime is not advisable. This can raise your cortisol and adrenaline levels. These stress hormones can keep you awake. It is recommended to exercise earlier in the day if at all possible, especially if you have sleeping problems. Exercises that I suggest you do before bedtime are yoga and stretching. Yoga might be able to calm your mind; therefore, it can help you to sleep better. Stretching can relieve muscle tension, which can also help your body to relax.

Try to have at least 30 minutes of quiet time before going to sleep, to let your mind calm down from the day's excitement and entertainment.

Get into the habit of listening to a guided meditation or adult bedtime story before bed to help your nervous system slow down and prepare your brain for sleep. Ideally, have it downloaded to your device so that you can turn off the screen and place it on aeroplane mode.

The more comfortable and relaxed you are before you try to sleep, the better the chances are that you are going to nod off quickly and stay that way until morning.

Avoid Eating Too Close to Bedtime

If your bedtime is 10 p.m., it is a good idea to have dinner no later than 7 p.m. if possible. It is no fun trying to sleep when you are bloated; you are more likely to stay awake, toss, and turn. I strongly suggest that you avoid eating for at least three hours before going to bed because this gives your body the chance to digest the food and prevents indigestion and stomach-ache. I also advise you not to drink anything an hour or two before going to bed. One of the most common reasons for disturbed sleep is having to use the toilet in the middle of the night and then not fall back asleep.

Avoid Caffeine and Alcohol

Drinking alcohol later at night is known to disrupt sleep patterns. It has been suggested to stop drinking caffeine at least six hours before you are ready to sleep.

Avoid anything containing caffeine or alcohol and instead opt for a warm, milky drink before you sleep or herbal tea such as chamomile. This will help relax you, making it easier for the dopamine to kick in (a hormone you need at this point), which helps you to sleep.

If you consume alcohol or caffeine:

- You are probably going to be up several times during the night to use the toilet.

- These are stimulants which will simply make you wide awake, rather than fast asleep.

- These can raise your blood sugar levels and negatively impact your sleep and overall health.

Never Take Your Phone to Bed with You

Having your phone underneath your pillow might seem practical, but it is a big distraction, as you are more likely to wake up whenever you hear a beep or feel a vibration.

Turn your phone off or put it on silent and keep it far away from your bed. If you are worried about oversleeping, set an old-fashioned alarm clock!

By having your phone next to you when you are trying to sleep, you are also more likely to start scrolling through social media, which will keep you awake.

Check the Temperature of Your Room

If your room is too hot or too cold, you will not find it easy to sleep properly. Try to adjust your room temperature so that it gets cooler at night, mimicking your body's natural temperature control. This increases melatonin production, which is a sleep hormone that tells your brain it is time to sleep. If the room is too hot or too stuffy, open a window or use a fan; if it is too cold, add some blankets rather than turning up the heating, which will just add to the stuffiness. You could also use an electric blanket, but do not sleep with it turned on all night; simply turn it on for an hour before you are going to sleep and then you will be warm and toasty.

Check Your Sleeping Environment

Aside from the temperature, check your bed and how comfortable it is. Does the mattress need turning? Do you need extra or fewer blankets? Is there something about the material of the blankets that bothers you? Are you allergic to feathers in the pillows?

Make sure your mattress is appropriate for your unique sleeping needs. Investing in a mattress that works for you can improve your sleep quality, so it is worth considering it. You should also check how long you have had your pillows for, as these do need to be changed regularly if you want them to be comfortable and supportive. A year or two is the maximum you should keep these.

Try a Weighted Blanket

Weighted blankets are regularly used to treat restless legs syndrome (RLS), but they are also useful for anyone who simply struggles with sleep. In this case, the blanket is heavier, and you can choose which weight you want it to be. The idea is that the blanket is like a hug, and as a result your body releases oxytocin, which is another hormone naturally occurring within the body. This hormone helps you relax and feel content, which is ideal for helping you get to sleep.

Keep a Pen and Paper Beside Your Bed

A good idea is to keep a pen and paper beside your bed. If you wake up with something you do not want to forget, scribble it down and work on it the next day. By simply writing it down, you have cast it from your mind and you will feel freer as a result. There is nothing more distracting when you are trying to sleep than remembering something and then feeling worried that you are going to forget it.

I find this tip very useful. As a writer, I always have lots of ideas going through my head. Not writing them down would prevent me from sleeping. Therefore, this works for me.

Try Lavender Oil

It goes without saying that you should check with your doctor if you have any problems, allergies, or taking any medications before trying any holistic or alternative therapies. If you are good to go, a lavender essential oil is a great go-to.

You could add a few drops to a warm bath before bed, try a pillow mist, or simply add a few drops to a tissue and leave it beside your pillow. Some people also find it useful to add a drop to the soles of their feet or their inner wrists, but in this case, you should water the oil down with a carrier oil, as undiluted essential oil can be damaging to the skin.

Lavender oil is known to relax and induce sleep while also being fantastic for anxiety and stress. Scents such as lavender, chamomile and sage have also been shown to have calming aromatic properties.

Sleep can help your body in so many ways. During this time, the body restores and rebalances itself. To achieve a good quality sleep it is vital to create the right environment, so your body can relax and you can have a good night's sleep. The number of hours you need to sleep every night depends on your individual needs.

Is Insomnia a Real Problem for You?

You might be confused about the difference between sleep deprivation and insomnia. The lines are quite blurred, but if you are struggling with sleep and nothing is making it better, you should certainly visit your doctor and discuss therapies or treatments which may improve your situation. Sleep deprivation over a long period, i.e. insomnia, is not something you should have to deal with.

If you are struggling with insomnia you will need to speak to your doctor about it. You will be asked a series of questions and perhaps even offered sleep studies to determine the cause. However, this is more likely to be the case if the problem is exceptionally prolonged or if you are suffering from other sleep-related issues, such as sleep apnea.

The bottom line is that if you are struggling with sleep, you need to make some lifestyle changes first and foremost and see if that makes a difference.

Many menopausal women find that their sleep is disturbed on and off throughout this time. It is not usually an ongoing and prolonged issue that drastically reduces your sleep, but if you are struggling and your life is affected by the lack of sleep, you need to get extra help to sort the problem out.

You might think that sleep is not important and that you are wasting your doctor's time, but you are not. Having a good night's sleep is crucial for many reasons. During this time your body gets a break from digesting the food and coping with stress. Remember that your body is the machine that never stops working. Sleep offers your body a chance to tidy up and restore, which reduces inflammation and supports healing.

Sleep is a vital part of your life, and it is something that your brain and body need in order to stay fit and healthy.

Of course, there is the weight gain side of the coin to consider too. Gaining weight due to the lack of sleep and subsequent unhealthy food choices means that you are also putting your health at risk. For all of these reasons, you need to make sleep a priority and work out how to make your situation better.

Key Points

In this chapter, I have talked about sleep and why the menopause may affect it. And we looked at the link between sleep and weight gain. The good news is that you can reverse this link by making some changes to your lifestyle, which will help you rectify your sleep problem.

The main points to remember from this chapter are:

- Sleep can be disturbed during the menopause.

- Sleep deprivation affects the levels of leptin and ghrelin within the body, which means that you are more likely to put on weight through unhealthy food choices.

- Hot flushes and night sweats can affect sleep, so you should try and remain as cool as possible and avoid hot drinks. Monitor the temperature of your room, and if necessary open the window.

- If you are struggling with insomnia, i.e. you are not sleeping well and are always tired during the day, you should see your doctor and find out what can help solve your problem.

- Most sleep problems can be solved or improved with a few changes to your lifestyle.

- Avoid overstimulating yourself before you sleep and look towards relaxation instead.

- You must go to bed and wake up at the same time every day, to ensure that your body clock remains regular and your hormones are therefore regulated far more easily.

- Progesterone is naturally lower during the menopause, and this is a hormone which is related to sleep.

- Sleep is a vital function for the brain and body, so never feel awkward or embarrassed to talk about it. During this time, your brain and your body are healing, regenerating, and getting ready for the next day. It is impossible to function effectively without sleep.

Chapter 7

Finding Support Around You

We are almost at the end of the book. I hope that you are feeling more hopeful and positive about the process that you are currently going through or anticipating. Because that is all it is: a process. Every process eventually comes to an end. Life continues either the same as before or enriched by the experience you have been through.

I sincerely hope that you will find the strength to deal with any difficulties that the menopause causes for you, and learn to see this time in your life as a transition, rather than a definition. I also hope the content in this book has helped you to realise that you can take control of your health, your weight, and your happiness, simply by choosing to take the right kind of action.

In this final chapter, I want to leave you feeling upbeat and positive. I want to give you a last inspiring talk to stay with you long after reading the final words, and I want to recap on the most important points you have learnt.

You do not have to go through the menopause alone. Some women do not want to share this deeply personal time in their life with others and that is perfectly fine, but some women would certainly benefit from talking a little more, sharing stories and perhaps learning coping mechanisms from other menopausal women.

My advice is to look to those around you for support if you feel you need it and travel through the menopause in a way which you think is best for you. There is no right or wrong answer. Go with what feels right.

The Menopause is Neither a Full Stop Nor a Definition

For some women, the most challenging part of the menopause is not the possible weight gain or the possible symptoms you might encounter, but what it stands for. The menopause is, as I have already outlined earlier in the book, the point at which you are no longer fertile; your menstrual cycle ends, and you move on to the next chapter of your life. In its very essence, that chapter does mean that you are moving into the second part of your life. And that is something that many women struggle to come to terms with.

It is all right to feel that way and you are certainly not alone. You need to realise that just because your menstrual cycle has finished and you are no longer releasing eggs to become pregnant, that does not make you any less of a woman. It simply means that your body is going through a cycle.

In many ways, the menopause makes you more of a woman than before, because you have earned your stripes. You have been there; you have done it. You have been through around 40 or so years of having periods every month. You have struggled with finding the right type of contraception and probably dealt with its side effects. You have battled with your hormones and won. You might have had children or maybe you did not, either way, it means that you have lived your fertile years as a woman. And you know what? You deserve to rest now. You deserve not to have to deal with a period every month, powerful contraceptive pills, menstrual cramps and the worry of pregnancy.

While the menopause can be difficult while you are going through it, and it can be a little up and down in the immediate years afterwards, everything will settle down, and you will feel better. This point in your life is not a full stop. It is not the end of anything; it simply means that your ovaries are not releasing eggs, but that should not have a significant impact on your daily life at this point. It is probably unlikely you will be thinking about having children at 50 anyway.

The menopause does not end anything and does not define your womanhood either. The other things in your life define you — your personality, confidence, passion, courage, intuition, kindness, the way you treat other people, the things you are good at, and the mark you leave on the world. Those are more important things to focus on than whether or not you are menstruating every month.

However, I can appreciate that the menopause can change the way a woman sees herself, especially when it comes to menopausal weight gain and how that affects confidence.

Any type of weight gain can be detrimental to confidence levels and when you are feeling low and not too great within yourself, it affects every single aspect of your life. You might start to notice a drop in your mood or become agitated with those around you or avoid social events because you worry about judgement on how you look. You might miss a great opportunity because you do not feel able to complete whatever it is you need to do.

We are always told that beauty is on the inside, and I agree entirely, but there is a lot of truth in the idea that how you feel about yourself is intrinsically tied to your outer appearance too.

My advice is this — make sure you follow the guidance in this book and focus on overall health and well-being. When you do that you really cannot go wrong in any way, you will be healthier, you will feel more energetic, you will be more upbeat, you will have more energy and your confidence levels will soar. Perhaps most pertinently, you will not gain weight because you have regained control over your body and those pesky hormones which create all sorts of problems during this time of your life.

It can be hard to resist temptation when your leptin and ghrelin hormones are totally out of sync, and you are hungry for seemingly no reason. But if you are following a healthy lifestyle, you will be stronger in your mind and feel less inclined to make poor food choices. Instead, you will reach for a snack that will not cause you to gain weight, grab a glass of water to fill you up, or go out for a walk to get some fresh air and therefore overcome the craving without any dietary damage.

The menopause is as much about how you approach it mentally as it is about how you deal with the symptoms on a physical level. Of course, there is a very emotional side to the menopause too, which also needs addressing. I want you to understand that the cycle you are going through now is simply part of life and not all of your life. You are not defined or judged on how you dealt with the menopause; nobody is going to talk about how difficult or otherwise you found the change. It is a personal deal that nobody else needs to be a part of unless you want them to be. However, as I will now further elaborate, seeking out support and sharing your feelings is a positive step to take.

Finding Support

As women, we can sometimes have a habit of knocking each other down, but in our more exceptional moments, we can also build each other up. If you reach out to someone to talk and admit that perhaps you are struggling and you need a little help, the chances are that they will be more than willing to lend you an ear, give you some advice and share their experiences. All you need to do is ask.

Some women do sail their way through the menopause without much stress or trouble, but those are in the minority. Many women struggle in some way, and the area in which you struggle is a personal thing.

Some women find that their biggest problem is a lack of sleep, while others cannot control their hunger, and that is massively contributing to their weight gain. Some cannot handle the hot flushes or night sweats, while others find the emotional side of the menopause more troublesome.

Tension or anxiety are common feelings experienced by many women when they reach the menopause. Whatever you are struggling with, I urge you to talk about it and be open about your experiences. By doing that, you are not only helping yourself, but you might also inspire other women who may be struggling and do not have the confidence within themselves to speak up and ask for help.

We live in a world of technology and while social media may be a double-edged sword in many ways, it does have its advantages. One of those aspects is the availability of support groups. Before the days of Facebook, we did not connect with those further away from us very easily. I am not suggesting that we have a smoother ride than women 30 or 40 years ago, but we do have a range of available resources that were unheard of in the past. We can use these resources and the availability of information to our benefit.

Search for Facebook support groups and be brave enough to discuss with other women the ways your body behaves and how you feel about those changes. In these groups, you will meet other like-minded women going through the same thing as you, and you never know, you might meet a new lifelong friend. These groups do not need to be all doom and gloom. You do not need to share your scare stories of hot flushes and night sweats, but you can talk about any aspects of the menopause you are struggling with and simply work through your issues with people who understand. You will find out about various ways to handle troublesome symptoms from other women in the group and probably feel better knowing that you have others by your side who support you.

You could also talk to your doctor and find out if the surgery is running any support groups, or whether they know of any community-based groups related to women's health. Most regional areas have such groups, and on the whole, you are unlikely to need to travel too far to find one.

If meeting strangers in this way is not for you, that is fine. You do not have to do this if you do not feel comfortable with it. In this case, make sure that you make time for friends and focus on your social life. By doing this, you are taking your mind off the troubles you might be going through, increasing your confidence in the process. Spending time with friends, laughing, having shared experiences and simply being in the presence of those we enjoy spending time with can be therapy in itself.

You can suggest some of the healthy lifestyle tips I mentioned throughout the book, like going to an exercise class together or perhaps just taking the dogs for a walk and having a chat as you do so.

A big part of dealing with the menopause healthily, avoiding weight gain and feeling confident within yourself is handling the emotional and mental aspects of the process.

The Power of Talking

It is good to talk, right? We are told to talk about how we feel because offloading emotions and problems can help put them into perspective, and the phrase "A problem shared is a problem halved" is true. In this case, you can talk to someone about how you are feeling, without judgement, and you will probably feel 10 times better afterwards. They do not even need to reply in some cases, simply saying the words out loud can be enough.

However, what do you do if you do not want to verbalise how you are feeling to another person?

In that case, start writing a journal. I mentioned journaling a little earlier when talking about food and exercise, but this is a different type of journal. Previously, I spoke about making a record to look for patterns, but the kind of journaling that I am referring to now is a way of getting your feelings out and feeling better for it. You do not have to show anyone this journal. It can be for your eyes only, but if you want to explain to someone how you feel but struggling to find the right words, you could simply pour your heart out on a piece of paper and give it to them instead.

You see, writing is cathartic. It is a way of looking through your feelings and making sense of what is going on inside your mind and within your heart. For the most part, simply writing down your thoughts and feelings can be enough of a release to help you handle the problem more healthily from that point onwards. However, if you feel like you would like another person's input, you simply need to find a person you trust — someone who understands.

There are many worries and concerns which may go through the mind of a menopausal woman. Some women might worry about changes in their appearance and feel concerned about their weight gain or the sudden appearance of wrinkles on their faces due to the low level of oestrogen.

Other women feel emotional and confused about their menopausal symptoms — hot flushes, brain fog, anxiety, thinning hair and dry skin. You might feel anxious about what is going on inside you and wonder why you do not feel *yourself* anymore. If you allow all of this to bottle up, you will become stressed and risk damaging your mental health. It is vital that you talk things through, whether you believe what you are saying is important or not. If it is bothering you, it is important. It is that simple.

Of course, during the menopause, it is not unusual for a woman to experience mood swings and to become agitated for no reason and perhaps to snap or shout at their nearest and dearest. You can blame your hormones for this, but your family and friends might not realise it and could take it quite personally. These outbursts result from the maelstrom of emotions and feelings you are experiencing because your hormones are dictating your every move at this point. But during your calmer moments — and you will have many of these — I suggest you sit down with your loved ones and talk about what is going on and how you feel.

By doing this, they will understand better. They will perhaps make some concessions for any further outbursts in the future, learn how not to take it personally and not become hurt by you snapping at them for no reason, and you will feel more supported as a result. In this case, the menopause could bring you closer to those around you, but it hinges on your ability to talk about it first and foremost. This is not a taboo subject; it happens to every woman on the planet — nobody gets to escape it. The menopause is a normal part of life and we should feel able to talk about what is going on and how we feel about the symptoms we experience, without worries over judgement or embarrassment.

Do not block out the people around you. Embrace their support and let them in. They are probably wondering what is going on with you, worrying why you are acting a little differently, or why you seem distracted or down. Talk about it, let them in, allow them to help. Even if they cannot practically help you and take it all away from you, simply talking about it candidly will help you and indirectly, help them.

The Menopause Does Not Last Forever

If there is one message I want to give you at this point, it is the reassurance that this is just a phase in your life and that the menopause does not and is not going to last forever. Sure, when you are lying awake at night suffering from a night sweat, you are probably wondering whether it is ever going to end. When you notice that your trousers are becoming a little tighter and it starts to make you question your appearance, you will wonder what happens and what is about to happen, but remember this — you have control.

The menopause will end, and your symptoms will eventually subside and leave you feeling normal again, whatever that may be. You will also feel yourself once more and are going to have the same — if not better — outlook on life.

I know, it does not seem that way at the moment. You are stressed, tired, confused and probably hungry, but if you follow the advice I have talked you through, you will find your menopausal experience to be far more positive and even uplifting than you could have imagined, before you picked up this book. Once it is all over, you will be healthier as a result.

Remember, the menopause does not last forever; this is just a small part of your life that you are living right now.

The postmenopausal stage has its challenges, but menopausal symptoms will gradually disappear. You can be healthy and feel good about your body despite your biological age. Your health and the quality of life in your later years will depend on the way you live right now. If you focus on self-care, eating healthily and living a healthy lifestyle, you will have a higher chance of enjoying your midlife and beyond.

Take Control of Your Health and Control Your Life

Finally, I want to mention that you have control here. It might seem like your hormones are in control, and to a certain degree they are, but those reins can be totally in your hands if you make the right choices. Choosing how you will live your life and what you are going to eat, how often you are going to exercise, who you are going to spend your time with, how much you are going to allow unfortunate circumstances to affect you, is totally in your control. Understanding this and accepting this challenge will bring incredible changes in your life.

You cannot change the fact that your body is changing as we speak. You cannot change the fact that you are moving towards a point in your life when you will not be ovulating or menstruating anymore. You cannot change the fact that you are becoming a little older. However, you can control any potential weight gain and you can control how you feel. You can do a lot to minimise most of your symptoms too. That puts you firmly in the driver's seat to decide how your menopausal journey goes.

Focusing on consuming foods that nourish your body, exercising regularly and finding activities that you love doing, will help you turn the menopause into a positive experience. By doing this, you are taking control of your life and that will feel fantastic. Of course, you do not need to be going through the menopause to do this, but what a great excuse!

Being kind to yourself and taking care of your body is a valuable experience and it is a gift that only you can give to yourself. This experience is something that you can learn a lot from, and you will also learn a lot about yourself and your needs throughout the entire process. Remember, you are in charge and your behavior will determine how well and healthy you are going to be. You cannot rely on other people to take care of your body. You need to take responsibility and do the best you can in order to give yourself a chance to feel well, look good and be proud of yourself.

By acting this way, you are going to be the healthiest you have ever been. Does this idea not make you feel excited? Does it not make you feel eager to get started?

Key Points

I hope that by the end of this chapter, you feel better about the changes you are experiencing in your life right now. Have some faith that this will not be forever and it is simply a stage in your life that you have to go through. Do you remember the time when you got your first period? Can you remember how scary and weird it all felt? Can you remember how everything felt like it was changing for a while afterwards?

Well, in some ways the menopause is a little like that, but the opposite situation. Rather than beginning your fertility journey, it has now come to an end. However, that does not need to be a full stop on your journey as a woman; it is simply a part of your life. The menopause does not have to be any kind of ending, but the beginning of a new life cycle.

Here are the main points to take from this chapter:

- The menopause does not last forever; what you are feeling now will end.

- Finding support from other women going through the same experiences as you can help you boost your confidence and give you a sounding board when you are struggling with a problematic symptom or with general worries and concerns.

- Search online for communities of people to talk to. You can also look for community groups in your local area.

- Meeting other women going or having gone through the menopause will help you build up your confidence and give your life a social boost.

- Do not shut out your family and friends. They may be worried about why you are agitated or struggling. Talk it out.

- Journaling can be a very cathartic way to deal with your emotions at this time.

- You have control over the situation and can control your health and weight.

- By focusing on your health and well-being, you will come out of the menopause far healthier than when you went into it.

Conclusion

And there we have it!

We have now reached the end of the book, and by this point, I hope you are feeling uplifted and more positive than you were at the beginning.

The menopause comes to all women. There is no escaping or avoiding it, but you can navigate your way through it and emerge with a smile on your face and a super-positive attitude.

I have said it before — the menopause does not define you as a woman. It does not give any value or take it away, it merely is a process which we all go through at this time in our lives and may cause some discomfort for some time. It is important to remember that you CAN handle this, just as you have handled everything else that life has thrown at you so far.

Add the menopause to your list of experiences which made you much stronger, because I promise you, by focusing on your health and well-being and learning to develop a more positive mindset, you will not waste one second of your time. There is no better way to react to a life change which may otherwise plunge you into the depths of worry and anxiety.

The main focus of this book is to help you avoid, lose and deal with menopausal weight gain. This is one of the most common effects of the menopause and it can be extremely challenging to deal with. Not only are you trying to handle all the other symptoms that are coming your way, but you are now noticing that your clothes are tighter and your body is changing shape. This has a way of knocking your self-confidence as well as changing the way you see yourself in the mirror.

Your weight does not define you either, but if you are a healthy weight and you like the way you look, your confidence will soar. Life is so much better when we are confident and happy with ourselves. That does not mean we need to be super-skinny; it means we need to be happy and healthy, that is it.

The advice I have given you in this book is all focused towards managing menopausal weight gain whilst handling the other symptoms. Many menopausal symptoms tend to wind into each other, such as sleep deprivation causing weight gain and mood changes. Low mood can affect weight gain because it is far easier to reach for something high in sugar when you are feeling down. Hormones can make you put on weight, but they can also affect your sleep and mood. The symptoms cause a vicious cycle, and this needs addressing. When you do that, you will notice benefits in various parts of your life no matter what your sole aim is.

By focusing on your health and well-being, you can make positive changes and dedicate yourself to leading a healthy lifestyle rather than following a random fad diet that is far too restrictive to be successful or manageable. You will notice that you will lose weight, feel great, have more energy, sleep better and feel more confident because of it. Therefore, the menopause could be the best time of your life if you allow it, and not a time which is entirely at the mercy of unrelenting hormones.

All that is left for me to do now is to wish you good luck. Be sure to take in every single piece of advice I have given you and please do not discount the idea of reaching out to other women going through the same experiences as you.

People around you can offer you plenty of safety, support and comfort. You should not have to deal with any challenging experience in life alone.

Our lives as women mean a constant change of events which lead towards a new life cycle. You are born, you release your first egg and start to menstruate, you have a monthly period for 30 or more years, you may have children, you may not, and then — just like that — Mother Nature decides that you have become too comfortable and she shakes things up a little.

When the storm is over, because at times it may feel like a storm, you will look back and be glad that you focused on the positive elements and protected your health for the many fun-filled years you have ahead of you.

I have given you a lot of information, but if you take anything from this book, I want it to be these key points:

- The menopause is the point at which you stop ovulating and stop releasing eggs.

- The period before the menopause begins is called the perimenopause. During this time, you may notice some symptoms, including irregular, light, or heavy periods.

- The main symptoms of the menopause include weight gain, hot flushes, night sweats, irritability, trouble sleeping and fatigue.

- Weight gain during the menopause can be a very troublesome issue for many women. During this time, visceral fat around the mid-section and abdomen is gained and it can be harder to lose than before.

- Hormonal imbalance during menopause is causing many changes inside your body.

- Not sleeping well affects your weight and contributes to low mood, trouble concentrating, and an increased risk of developing severe health issues in later life. Focusing on sleep quality is vital.

- By making sensible life choices and deciding to focus on your health and well-being, you can overcome many menopausal symptoms and reduce menopausal weight gain as a direct consequence.

- To focus on your health, you need to have a balanced, healthy diet and be physically active.

- Like many women, you may feel less attractive while going through the menopause but focusing on your health will help restore your confidence and radiance.

- The menopause is not a full stop to your active years, it is simply a process that you are going through for a while before entering a different stage of life.

- Seek out help and support from other women going through the same thing as you and be sure to talk to your nearest and dearest too.

- The menopause will end. It is not a cycle that is always going to be in your life.

- Remember, you are a strong woman, you are a warrior and you have got this!

There is never a better time than now to make a fresh start and take control of your health and your life. Be nice to yourself — do not wait another moment!

I wish you all the best!

Lots of love xx

Silvana

Thank You

I hope you enjoyed this book!

Please consider leaving a review on Amazon – even if it is only a few sentences, it would be a huge help. Here is the link for your convenience. Go to http://viewbook.at/beat-menopause. Your review will help other readers benefit from the information in this book.

Please visit bit.ly/silvana-signup to join the mailing list for updates on future books and to receive information about health, weight loss, and nutrition.

About the Author

Silvana Siskov has spent more than 20 years working with people experiencing a variety of issues, such as mental health, eating disorders and weight management problems. Her main speciality is giving sound advice with a strong focus on emotional support. She is also dedicated to helping clients find a strong direction in the areas of their lives where they need it the most.

Silvana helps establish clarity around the issues which her clients are facing in their everyday lives. This allows them to take control over their health and well-being and change their lifestyle towards the positive end of the scale. By doing this, they are able to achieve their health goals and improve their confidence levels and sense of self-worth.

Following some personal health issues, Silvana's interest in nutrition grew. This led her towards supporting clients on their weight loss journeys, giving them advice on nutrition and their dietary needs and helping them overcome pitfalls such as comfort eating.

From this experience, *Get Your Sparkle Back: 10 Steps to Weight Loss and Overcoming Emotional Eating* was born. The fantastic reaction to this book led her to write more, helping her clients achieve their lifestyle goals and feel more confident from within. *Live Healthy on a Tight Schedule* quickly followed suit, empowering readers to be far less dependent on external factors and to take more control of their lives.

Shortly after this book was published, the book *Get Fit and Healthy in Your Own Home in 20 Minutes or Less* was written. This book continues to help Silvana's readers to work towards their health and weight loss goals.

Silvana finds true pleasure in supporting her clients and working closely with them on a one-on-one basis. She also extends her work into the community, with talks and workshops for those who prefer a more sociable atmosphere.

Silvana's overall mission is to empower and motivate women, helping them to use their power from within and create a deeper connection to themselves. By doing so, they can achieve whatever they put their minds to, living their very best lives.

Helpful Resources

Books by Silvana Siskov:

- *"Get Your Sparkle Back: 10 Steps to Weight Loss and Overcoming Emotional Eating."* The book is available on Amazon. Go to http://viewbook.at/sparkle.

- *"Live Healthy on a Tight Schedule: 5 Easy Ways for Busy People to Develop Sustainable Habits Around Food, Exercise and Self-Care."* The book is available on Amazon. Go to http://viewbook.at/livehealthy.

- *"Get Fit and Healthy in Your Own Home in 20 Minutes or Less: An Essential Daily Exercise Plan and Simple Meal Ideas to Lose Weight and Get the Body You Want."* The book is available on Amazon. Go to http://viewbook.at/get-fit.

- *"Get Fit and Healthy on a Tight Schedule 2 Books in 1."* The book is available on Amazon. Go to http://viewbook.at/get-fit2books.

- *"Free Yourself From Hot Flushes and Night Sweats: The Essential Guide to a Happy And Healthy Menopause."* The book is available on Amazon. Go to http://viewbook.at/healthy-menopause.

- *"Break the Binge Eating Cycle: Stop Self-Sabotage and Improve Your Relationship With Food."* The book is available on Amazon. Go to http://viewbook.at/breakthebinge.

- *"Relaxation and Stress Management Made Simple: 7 Proven Strategies to Calm Your Mind, Stop Negative Thinking and Improve Your Life."* The book is available on Amazon. Go to http://viewbook.at/stressfree.

Free Mini-Courses:

- *Discover 10 Secrets of Successful Weight Loss*

- *This is How to Start Eating Less Sugar*

- *Learn How to Boost Your Energy – 11 Easy Ways*

- *Your Guide to a Happy and Healthy Menopause*

- *This is How to Lose Weight in Your 40s and Beyond*

Free Mini-Courses Available at:

www.silvanahealthandnutrition.com/course/